Complications in Orthopaedics
Distal Radius Fractures

D1796687

Edited by
Steven L. Friedman, MD
Hand and Upper Extremity Surgery
Orthopaedic Specialty Center
Baltimore, Maryland

Series Editor
Jeffrey O. Anglen, MD
Indiana University Medical Center
Indianapolis, Indiana

Published by the
American Academy of Orthopaedic Surgeons
6300 North River Road
Rosemont, IL 60018

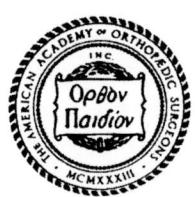

American Academy of Orthopaedic Surgeons

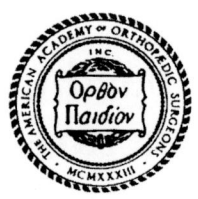

The material presented in *Distal Radius Fractures* has been made available by the American Academy of Orthopaedic Surgeons for educational purposes only. This material is not intended to present the only, or necessarily best, methods or procedures for the medical situations discussed, but rather is intended to represent an approach, view, statement, or opinion of the author(s) or producer(s), which may be helpful to others who face similar situations.

Some drugs or medical devices demonstrated in Academy courses or described in Academy print or electronic publications have not been cleared by the Food and Drug Administration (FDA) or have been cleared for specific uses only. The FDA has stated that it is the responsibility of the physician to determine the FDA clearance status of each drug or device he or she wishes to use in clinical practice.

PMMA bone cement is considered a device for FDA purposes. In October 1999, the FDA reclassified PMMA bone cement as a Class II device for its intended use "in arthroplastic procedures of the hip, knee and other joints for the fixation of polymer or metallic prosthetic implants to living bone." The use of a device for other than its FDA-cleared indication is an off-label use. Physicians may use a device off-label if they believe, in their best medical judgment, that its use is appropriate for a particular patient (eg, tumors).

Furthermore, any statements about commercial products are solely the opinion(s) of the author(s) and do not represent an Academy endorsement or evaluation of these products. These statements may not be used in advertising or for any commercial purpose.

Some of the authors or the departments with which they are affiliated have received something of value from a commercial or other party related directly or indirectly to the subject of their chapter.

First Edition
Copyright 2005 by the
American Academy of Orthopaedic Surgeons

ISBN 0-89203-367-3

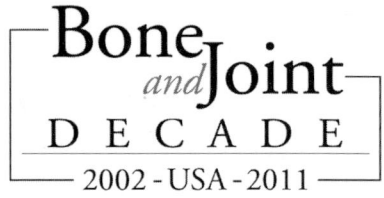

Contributors

Steven L. Friedman, MD
Hand and Upper Extremity Surgery
Orthopaedic Specialty Center
Baltimore, Maryland

Brian Harley, MD
SUNY Upstate Medical University
Syracuse, New York

F. Thomas D. Kaplan, MD
Indiana Hand Center
Indianapolis Indiana

Andrew K. Palmer, MD
Director of Hand Surgery
Professor of Orthopaedic Surgery
Department of Orthopaedics
Upstate Medical University
Syracuse, New York

Peter J. Ronchetti, MD
Clinical Assistant Professor of Orthopaedic Surgery
University of Rochester
Rochester, New York

Colby R. Young, MD
Hand Associates of the Nevada Desert, LLC
Las Vegas, Nevada

Contents

Preface

Most fractures encountered in the United States affect the upper extremity, and the most common of these are fractures of the distal radius. Many excellent publications focus on the evaluation and management of the wide spectrum of possible injuries to the wrist, in general, and distal radius fractures, in particular. However, surprisingly little has been published that focuses on complications arising from distal radius fractures. This monograph addresses, in a case presentation format, the recognition, prevention, and management of such complications.

The upper extremity is the anatomic structure through which individuals physically interact with their environment, placing the hand and wrist at constant risk of injury. Most distal radius fractures are relatively innocuous injuries that are satisfactorily treated by cast or splint immobilization. Nonetheless, a significant number of these fractures result in serious long-term morbidity. The mechanism of injury is the primary determining factor of long-term outcome and frequency of complications in these injuries. Complications generally can be grouped as those related to the injury and those related to treatment and can be further categorized based on the anatomic structures affected. In this monograph, a number of respected upper extremity orthopaedic specialists address complications of distal radius fractures, including malunions, nonunions, injuries to the distal radioulnar joint (DRUJ), contractures, neurologic injuries and complex regional pain syndrome (CRPS), hardware issues, and other related injuries. In these times of increasing medical malpractice awareness and litigation, it is important for all orthopaedic surgeons to be cognizant of the potential for complications, particularly in these very commonly encountered fractures.

Malunions of the distal radius, which are among the most commonly encountered problems, frequently occur in the elderly population but may be seen in pediatric and adult patients, particularly after high-energy trauma. Malunions can occur following surgical or nonsurgical treatment and typically result in loss of radial height and of ulnar and volar inclination of the articular surface of the distal radius. Although less common, intra-articular malunions can result in loss of articular congruity. In addition to cosmetic deformity, malunited fractures may lead to problems with midcarpal instability, ulnar impaction syndrome, radiocarpal arthritis, and distal radioulnar joint arthritis or instability.

Nonunions are particularly uncommon because most distal radius fractures affect the metaphyseal portion of the distal radius, which tends to heal promptly. High-energy injuries and excessive soft tissue stripping associated with combined volar and dorsal internal fixation increase the risk of nonunion as a result of devascularization. Inadequate immobilization, often caused by noncompliance, can also increase the risk of nonunion as can deep infection and peripheral neuropathy. Nonunion generally requires surgical intervention because of the associated pain, deformity, and dysfunction.

Fractures of the distal radius frequently affect the congruity and function of the DRUJ. Tears of the triangular fibrocartilage complex can lead to pain or DRUJ instability, and fractures compromising the integrity of the sigmoid notch and certain fractures of the ulnar styloid also can cause DRUJ instability. Intra-articular fractures affecting the sigmoid notch also can lead to DRUJ arthritis. Furthermore, surgical implants about the wrist can impact on the function of the DRUJ and extensor carpi ulnaris tendon.

The hand and wrist are particularly vulnerable to contractures and joint stiffness because of the importance of mobility to hand function. Stiffness and contractures in the fingers and wrist can result from closed or open treatment of distal radius fractures; however, a common cause of these problems is the use of external fixation that depends on longitudinal distraction that bridges multiple articulations. Hand function can be compromised seriously by stiffness, leading to the possibility of the cure being more debilitating than the disease in some cases.

Neurologic injury and CRPS are commonly seen in association with distal radius fractures. The median nerve usually is involved, yet injury to the ulnar and radial nerves also can be seen. Nerve injury can be a consequence of the injury itself or of surgical fixation. Compartment syndrome, another concern in high-energy injuries or those involving anticoagulation, must be rapidly diagnosed and treated to avoid permanent functional compromise. CRPS also benefits from prompt recognition and treatment, although a delay in diagnosis tends to occur in a large number of patients. CRPS, nerve injury, and compartment syndrome may lead to severe functional compromise and, in some patients, chronic pain if a significant delay in treatment occurs.

With advances in technology, the role for surgical intervention in the treatment of distal radius fractures and recognition of problems related to surgical fixation have grown. External fixation has a relatively high association with complications, including pin tract infection, overdistraction, radial sensory nerve injury, and pin-associated fractures. Complications of internal fixation implants include loss of fixation, articular compromise, material failure, and problems associated with extensor tendon irritation or attrition. Each of these obstacles can compromise the outcome of a properly treated fracture.

This list of complications illustrates the inherently hazardous nature of evaluating and treating fractures of the distal radius. It is difficult for surgeons to frankly discuss complications and errors in diagnosis and treatment. Consequently, there is a paucity of printed material addressing this important subject. I believe that this frank discussion of complications will improve the overall quality of care provided to those who place their confidence in orthopaedic surgeons, and I sincerely hope that orthopaedic surgeons will find this monograph valuable.

I would like to thank the contributors to this monograph for their time and effort, and I want to thank the AAOS Publications Department for their input and the work to bring this project to fruition.

Steven L. Friedman
Editor

MALUNION

Brian J. Harley, MD, FRCSC
Andrew K. Palmer, MD

CASE PRESENTATION

A 38-year-old woman presented to the emergency department after falling on her nondominant, outstretched left arm while coming down a short flight of stairs. She reported pain in the left wrist and had an obvious deformity. She denied any prior history of wrist injury and noted no numbness or tingling in her fingers. The patient was otherwise healthy and worked as a legal aide. Physical examination revealed significant deformity at the left wrist with swelling and tenderness. Her fingers were well perfused but had poor mobility because of pain. Radiographs obtained in the emergency department showed a dorsally displaced and tilted distal radius fracture (**Figure 1,** *A* and *B*).

The patient consented to a closed reduction under sedation in the emergency department, and a sugar-tong splint was applied. Postreduction radiographs were obtained, and the treating physician felt that an acceptable reduction had been obtained (**Figure1,** *C*). However, the casting material prevented clear visualization of the reduction, and the wax pencil mark on the lateral view represented the treating physician's impression of the postreduction lateral tilt (**Figure 1,** *D*). Unfortunately, the line bisects the dorsal radius with the volar ulnar head and underestimates the actual deformity on the lateral view.

The patient was seen in the office 2 weeks later and placed into a long arm cast. Radiographs in the cast were obtained at this time (**Figure 1,** *E* and *F*). Once again, the views were less than ideal; a very oblique lateral view was obtained. Despite the poor lateral view, it appears that the distal fragment fell back into a dorsally tilted position, very much like the radiographs obtained at presentation. The position in the cast was accepted, and the patient returned 6 weeks later for cast removal. At that time, she was placed in a removable wrist brace for support, and an outpatient physical therapy program was initiated with the goal of improving range of motion (ROM) and function. She was reassured that she would "do well" despite the obvious cosmetic deformity in her wrist.

As soon as the physical therapy regimen began, the patient reported increasing numbness and tingling in her hand, especially with activity. Although she noted a fairly rapid improvement in motion in the first 6 weeks, full ROM was not restored, especially wrist flexion and radial deviation. She described a heavy feeling in her fingers and difficulty with fine motor activities such as applying

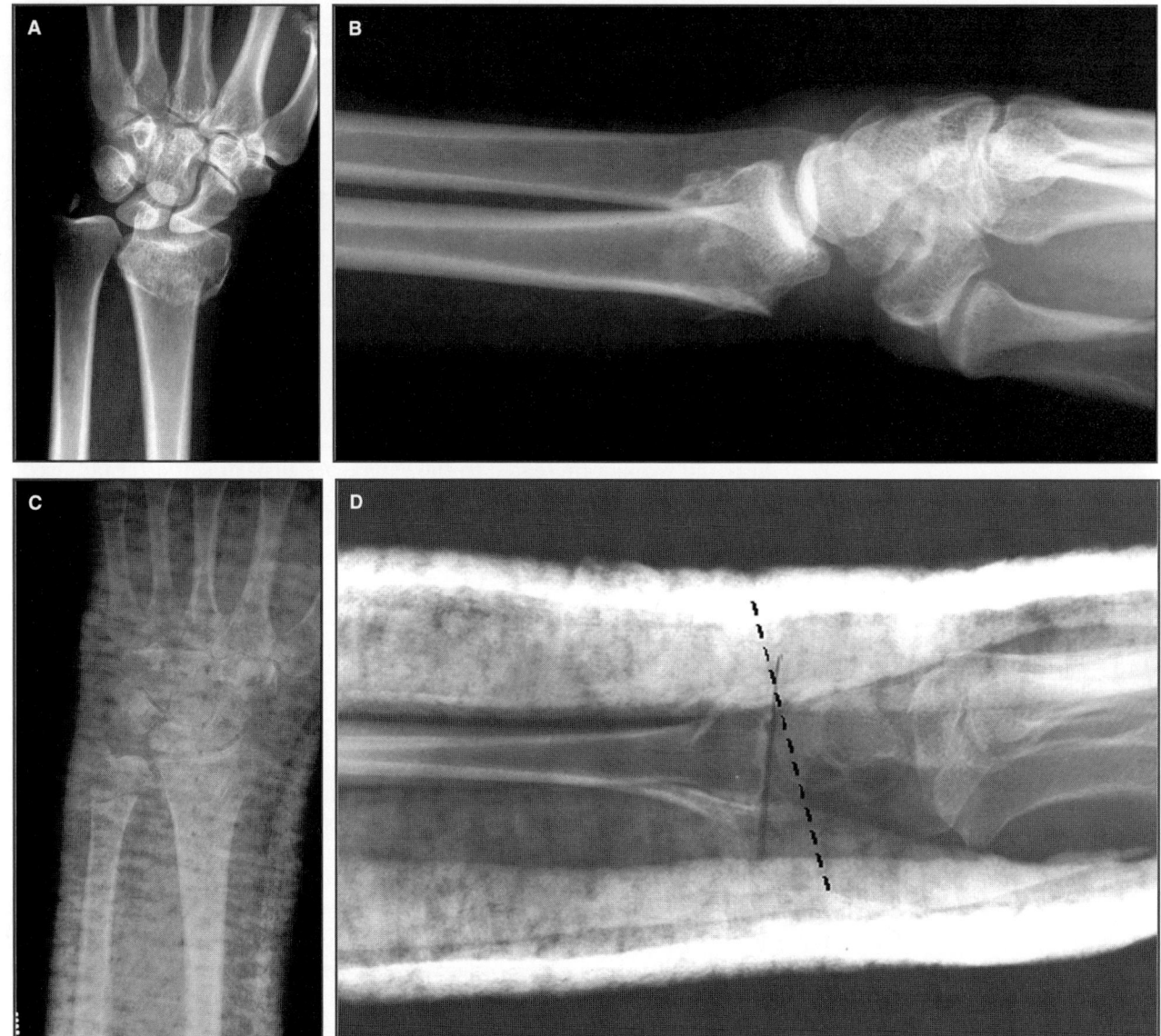

Figure 1 A, Initial PA radiograph reveals increased ulnar variance and loss of radial inclination. **B,** Initial lateral view reveals dorsal tilt and dorsal comminution. **C,** Postreduction PA view reveals improved alignment. **D,** The postreduction lateral view reveals a failure to obtain neutral tilt. The wax pencil line represents the treating physician's initial assessment of volar tilt, incorrectly defining a line between the dorsal radial articular margin and the volar margin of the ulnar head and, thereby, underestimating the actual dorsal tilt. The real volar tilt is marked by the hatched line.

makeup, doing her hair, and using a computer keyboard. Most problematic was that even 6 months after the injury, she noted persistent wrist pain, both dorsally and ulnarly, that prevented her from performing her duties at work. She was motivated to do

whatever was necessary to improve function and reduce the wrist pain.

Examination at 6 months revealed an obvious deformity, with a radially deviated hand and a prominent distal ulna (**Figure 2,** *A* and *B*). ROM was de-

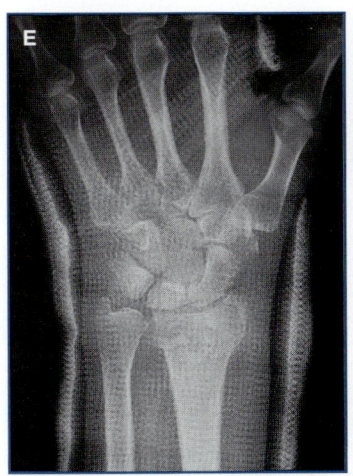
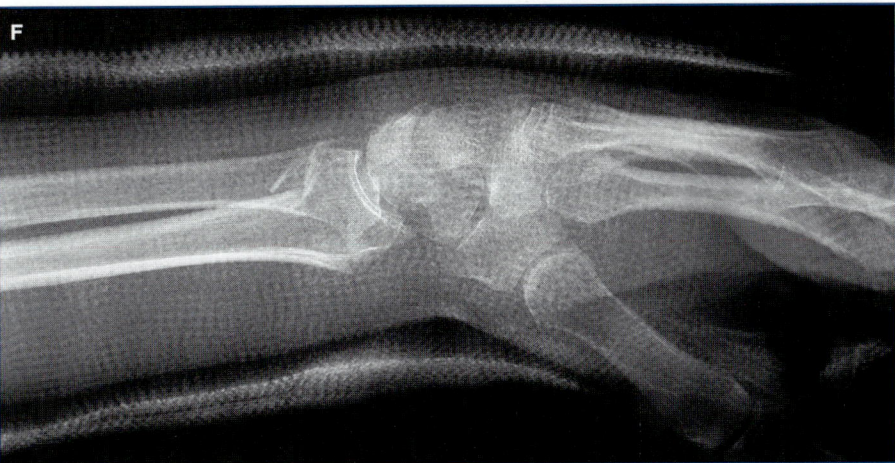

Figure 1 (continued) PA **(E)** and lateral **(F)** radiographs in a cast 2 weeks after reduction reveal loss of the reduction such that the fracture closely resembles the initial radiographs.

creased in all directions compared with the opposite wrist, with flexion most restricted. The patient had a withdrawal response with passive motion and tenderness to palpation at the ulnar head. The distal radioulnar joint (DRUJ) was less stable than in the opposite normal wrist but not dislocatable. Thenar strength was normal, but she reported decreased sensation in the thumb, index, and middle fingers.

Radiographs obtained at this time reveal an obvious distal radius malunion (**Figure 2,** *C* and *D*). The radiographs also show increased ulnar variance compared with the opposite, normal wrist (**Figure 2,** *E*), loss of radial inclination, and nearly 35° of dorsal tilt. The surface of the radiocarpal joint appears well aligned, and there are no obvious signs of joint degeneration. The ulnar styloid is intact; however, a small subchondral cyst is evident on the ulnar aspect of the proximal lunate. Carpal alignment reveals an early compensatory midcarpal flexion of the capitate and scaphoid on the lunate.

DISCUSSION

Wrist fractures are among the most commonly treated musculoskeletal problems. At one time, closed reduction and casting was the only viable treatment, frequently resulting in malunion. With the improvements in external and internal fixation techniques over the last 25 years, the approach to these fractures

has become much more aggressive. Nonetheless, this fracture is so common that malunion continues to be seen in the clinical setting. These same innovations in orthopaedic technology also can be used in the treatment of malunions. From imaging to small fragment fixation to bone graft substitutes, all facets of the treatment of this challenging clinical condition continue to change. Today's surgeon needs a keen grasp of anatomy, clinical examination, the latest techniques (those that have been proved clinically effective), and a thorough understanding of the indications for and the expected results of treatment before undertaking the surgical correction of a wrist malunion.

Evaluation of a Malunion
Clinical Assessment

Historically, almost all wrist fractures were believed to eventually heal acceptably. A wealth of basic science and clinical studies in the last century suggests that wrist fracture malunion can result in significant disability.[1-9] Pain, impaired motion, midcarpal instability, ulnar impaction, unacceptable cosmesis, and joint degeneration are frequent outcomes of malunion and are commonly seen.

These same symptoms, however, often occur in patients with a well-aligned and healing wrist fracture. Most patients obtain only 80% to 85% of their normal motion and strength after a well-aligned fracture

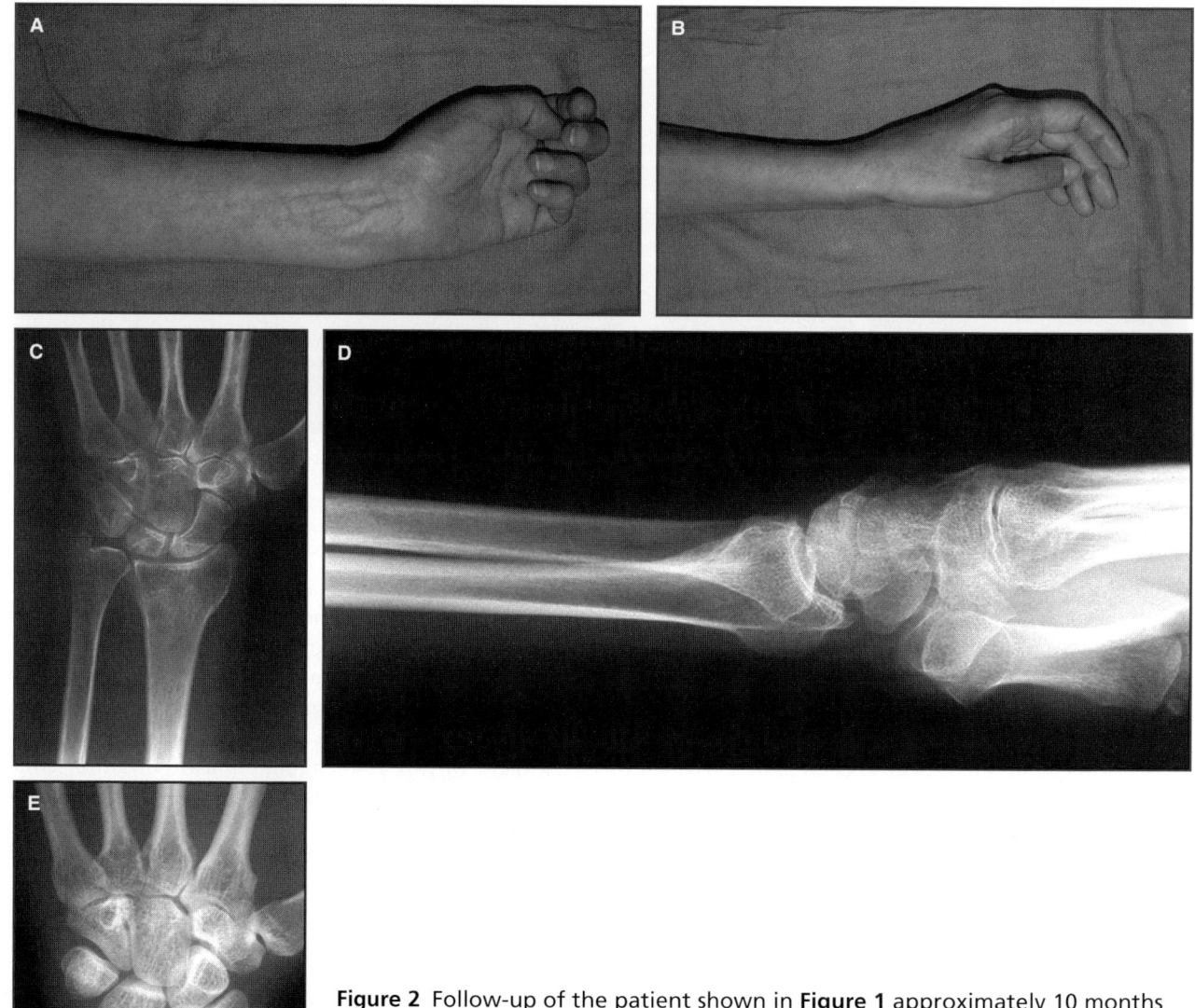

Figure 2 Follow-up of the patient shown in **Figure 1** approximately 10 months after the distal radius fracture. She reported global pain, decreased range of motion, and deformity. Dorsal **(A)** and volar **(B)** clinical photographs reveal radial deviation and a prominent ulnar head. PA **(C)** and lateral **(D)** radiographs reveal shortening, loss of radial inclination, and dorsal tilt of 40° with adaptive carpal alignment. **E,** Comparative PA view of the opposite normal wrist reveals neutral ulnar variance.

heals. Many patients, especially those who sustain higher-energy mechanisms of injury, experience even poorer outcomes despite acceptable radiographic outcomes.[7,9] Studies of wrist fractures have shown consistent improvement in clinical outcomes up to, and perhaps even beyond, 1 year after fracture. Therefore, patients must be advised that pain and/or loss of motion that persists 4 to 8 months after a fracture may resolve with time. However, for a patient whose recovery has clearly plateaued at 1 year or more after fracture, careful assessment of symptoms and deformity often points to surgical correction of the malunion in an effort to improve clinical outcome.

Entrapment or rupture of tendons about the wrist

has been seen after wrist malunion, and deformity may be a cause of tendon attrition or inefficiency that accounts for loss of strength or function. Likewise, carpal tunnel symptoms and other neurologic symptoms may develop in association with wrist malunion. Many patients, who perhaps had subclinical symptoms before fracture, can present with an exacerbation of their symptoms as a result of the malunion. Last, disruption of the triangular fibrocartilage complex and/or intercarpal ligament injury can be a source of pain in patients with wrist malunions. Documentation of DRUJ stability is important to help guide surgical planning. Unfortunately, the significance of some of these associated injuries is much more difficult to assess in patients with altered wrist bone anatomy. By convention, symptoms or findings that could be attributed to these soft-tissue injuries are generally addressed after radial realignment surgery, which can significantly reduce symptoms in most patients.

Radiographic Assessment

Surgeons generally assess the bony alignment of malunions by means of radiographic parameters. The surgeon's focus may be limited to the bones themselves because bony alignment is relatively easily assessed on plain radiographs, and, historically, great attention has been paid to this radiographic feature. However, bony alignment represents only one part of the complex interaction that predicts normal wrist function; the complex ligamentous arrangements that hold the bones in close proximity are equally essential to normal wrist function. One reason to surgically realign a malunion is to restore soft-tissue balance and loading and ultimately improve wrist function.

The three most commonly described radiographic parameters are variably named throughout the literature. For the purpose of this chapter, the parameters are labeled as follows: radial inclination, volar tilt, and ulnar variance. Radial inclination defines the angle that the distal radial articular surface makes with the perpendicular to the shaft of the radius on a neutral rotation PA view (**Figure 3, A**). The distal radial articular surface is a line connecting the tip of the radial styloid with the ulnarmost base of the distal radius. The angle between this line and the perpendicular of the shaft of the radius generally is 22°.

Volar tilt defines the angle that the distal radial articular surface makes with a line perpendicular to the shaft of the radius on a neutral rotation lateral radiograph (**Figure 3, B**). On this view, the distal radial articular surface is a line connecting the dorsal articular lip to the volar articular lip. The angle between this line and the line perpendicular to the shaft of the radius generally measures between 10° and 11°.

Ulnar variance defines the distance between the distal radial articular surface and the seat of the distal ulna (**Figure 3, C**); it represents a measurement of the relationship between the distal ulna and the lunate facet of the distal radius on a PA radiograph. A comparative PA view of the uninjured wrist is essential because it is impossible to know the amount of shortening within a wrist malunion unless the true ulnar variance of the opposite, normal side is available for comparison.

Radiographs are the most useful way to assess bone alignment at the time of acute fracture, as well as before and after treatment of a malunion. However, those radiographs must be true PA and lateral views centered on the wrist joint. Rotated PA or lateral views can lead to poor perception of the true articular surface alignment. A pair of oblique views also can provide visualization of articular gaps or steps not easily visualized on the PA and lateral views. Before any surgical correction of a wrist malunion can be attempted, a clear understanding of the deformity is paramount. The four radiographic parameters that need to be determined prior to surgical treatment are (1) changes in angulation (in sagittal and coronal planes), (2) degree of shortening, (3) joint incongruity, and (4) rotational deformity.

Changes in Angulation

Angulation deformity should be assessed on both the PA and lateral radiographs. The most common condition is a dorsal tilt of the epiphyseal fragment. This deformity results from comminution of the dorsal metaphyseal surface combined with loading of adjacent tendons leading to collapse of the dorsal cortex. Clinical and basic science studies have documented the adverse effect of this dorsally tilted position in which increasing symptoms correlate with increasing deformity.[1,4-6,10,11] Although a volarly tilted or even a neutral position on the lateral view is preferred after fracture reduction and healing, corrective surgery for deformity with up to 10° to 15° of dorsal tilt generally

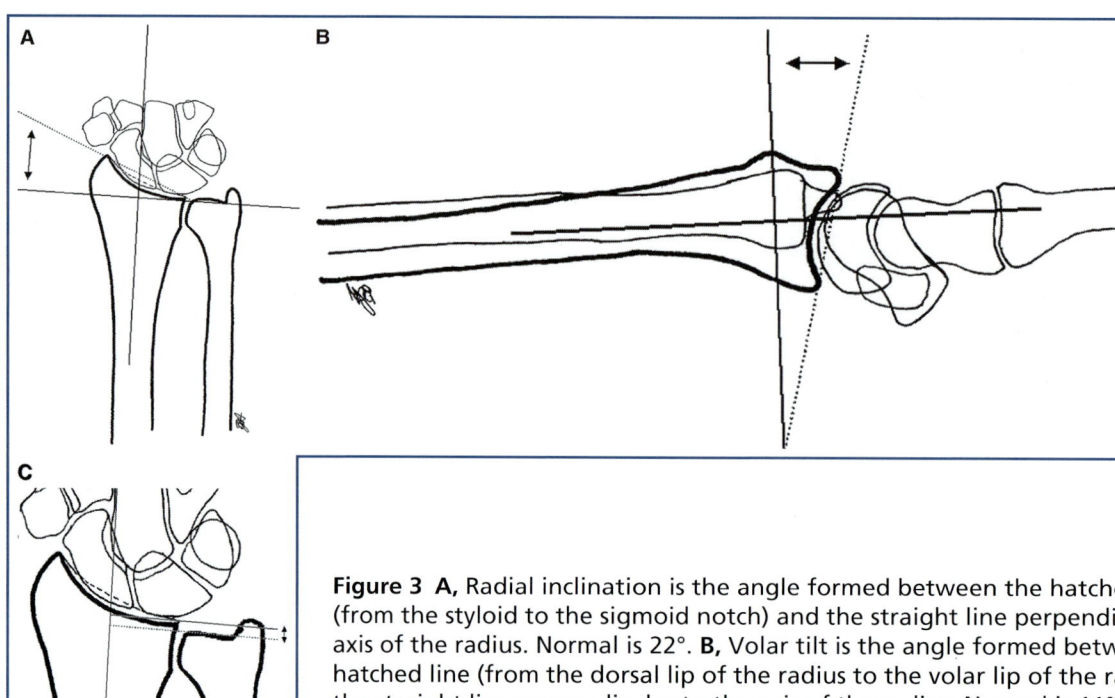

Figure 3 A, Radial inclination is the angle formed between the hatched line (from the styloid to the sigmoid notch) and the straight line perpendicular to the axis of the radius. Normal is 22°. **B,** Volar tilt is the angle formed between the hatched line (from the dorsal lip of the radius to the volar lip of the radius) and the straight line perpendicular to the axis of the radius. Normal is 11°. **C,** Ulnar variance is the distance in millimeters between the ulnar edge of the radial articular surface and the seat of the distal ulna. Normal varies for each person, and the opposite, normal wrist serves as the most reliable control in a patient with a wrist fracture.

is not advised. In fact, most studies report limited impairment in function with deformity of this lesser degree.[1,4,5,10] As the deformity increases beyond this level, however, and with the typical clinical symptoms, surgeons and patients tend to pursue surgical correction of the malunion.

Although volarly tilted malunions are significantly less common, they are believed to alter function and cause clinical symptoms (**Figure 4**). Typically, malunion occurs after a volarly displaced wrist fracture, but overreduction of a dorsally tilted radius fracture also is a possible cause. The radiographs must be carefully scrutinized for any volar subluxation of the carpal bones indicative of a volar Barton's fracture, which could necessitate an intra-articular corrective osteotomy. The extent of volar deformity that would require surgical correction has not been as clearly defined as the extent of dorsally tilted malunion. We believe that volar angulation more than 15° beyond normal (a minimum of 25° of total volar tilt), combined with clinical symptoms, constitute a reasonable indication for surgery.

Whether dorsally or volarly tilted on the lateral view, almost all malunions show loss of radial inclination on the PA view, likely the result of the pull of the brachioradialis tendon on the radial styloid. Isolated loss of the radial inclination with wrist malunion is uncommon, but the loss of inclination can cause significant clinical discomfort. Disability is generally seen with loss of radial inclination of 10° or more and is generally the result of a clinical loss of ulnar deviation combined with increased ulnar variance.

Shortening

Shortening after a wrist malunion also commonly causes pain, decreased ROM, and increased prominence of the distal ulna. In fact, shortening may be more disabling than angulation deformity. Radial shortening results from the comminution and loss of integrity of the cortical surfaces combined with the forces generated by the flexor and extensor tendons across the wrist joint. The natural relationship at the DRUJ becomes disrupted, and this disruption can lead

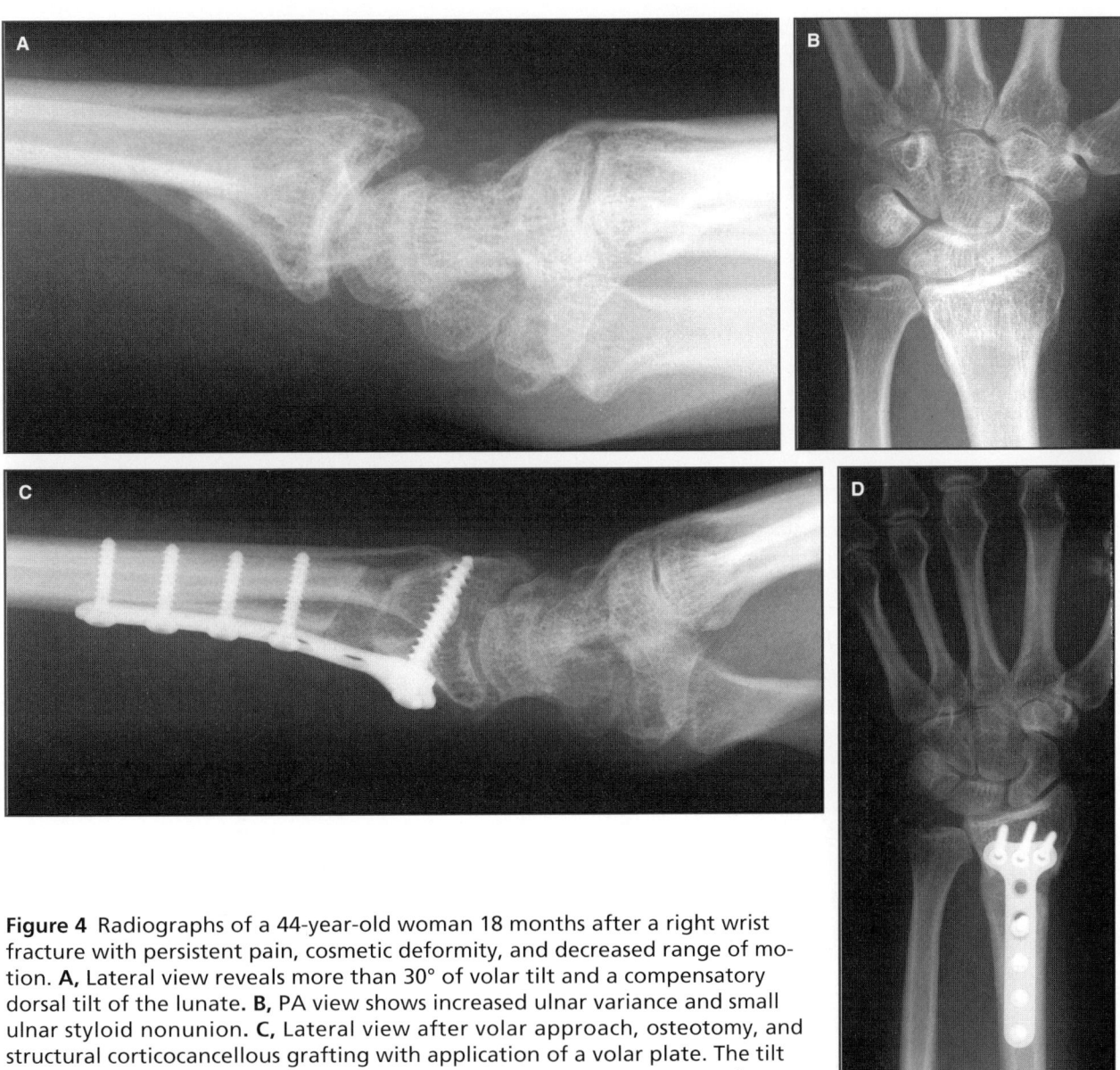

Figure 4 Radiographs of a 44-year-old woman 18 months after a right wrist fracture with persistent pain, cosmetic deformity, and decreased range of motion. **A,** Lateral view reveals more than 30° of volar tilt and a compensatory dorsal tilt of the lunate. **B,** PA view shows increased ulnar variance and small ulnar styloid nonunion. **C,** Lateral view after volar approach, osteotomy, and structural corticocancellous grafting with application of a volar plate. The tilt has been corrected to 15°. **D,** PA view after corrective osteotomy reveals correction of ulnar variance.

to either instability or stiffness. Furthermore, with proximal migration of the distal radial articular surface, an increasing proportion of the load across the wrist is transferred to the intact ulnar head and can result in symptoms typical of ulnar impaction.[8,12] Although evidence supports corrective osteotomy for as little as 2 mm of shortening, some patients can tolerate shortening up to 5 mm. A comparative PA radio-

graph of the opposite, normal wrist is essential to assess the natural ulnar variance and allow for accurate assessment of the amount of shortening.

Shortening can occur from a combination of both apparent and real loss of bone length (**Figure 5**). Apparent shortening results from dorsal comminution and the resultant tilting effect of the malunion. This effect is apparent because the volar cortex generally is

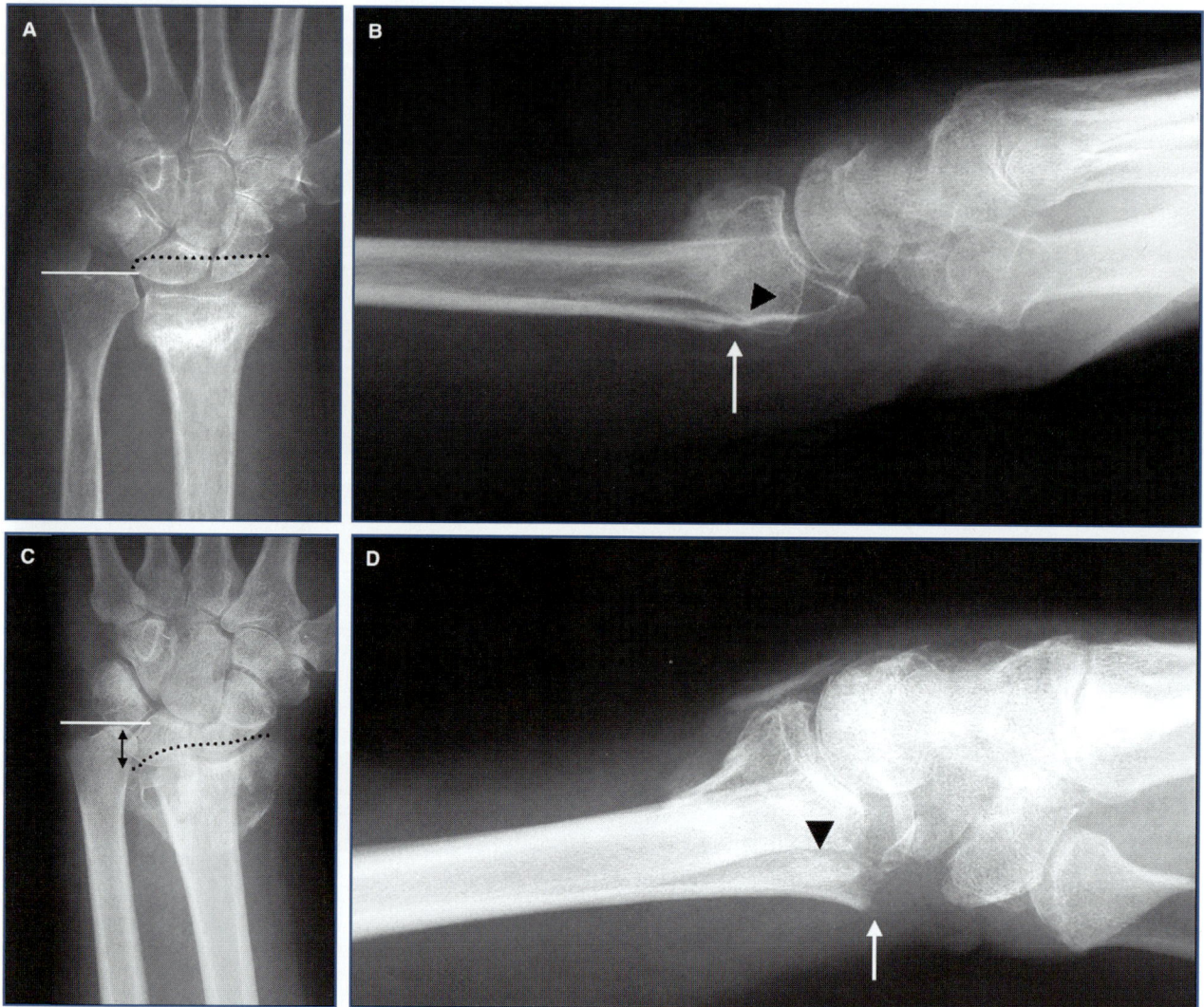

Figure 5 **A,** PA view of malunion with *apparent* positive ulnar variance. The outline of the volar rim of the distal radius (dotted line), however, reveals that the volar length of the radius has been maintained when measured against the ulnar head (white line). **B,** Lateral view reveals minimal shortening (arrow) and no volar step-off (arrowhead). This type of malunion is easily correctable with angular osteotomy, plating, and cancellous grafting. **C,** PA view of malunion with a *real* increase in ulnar variance. The dotted line on the volar rim reveals significant loss of length of volar rim (double arrow) when measured against the ulnar head (white line). **D,** Lateral view shows shortening (arrow) and volar step-off (arrowhead). Correcting the length of this type of malunion is difficult and typically requires a structural corticocancellous graft and rigid plating for support. This patient eventually required wrist arthrodesis because of the severe soft-tissue contractures that prevented anatomic restoration.

not shortened. In some malunions, the lateral radiograph clearly shows that volar length has been maintained. Real shortening results from the loss of length at both dorsal and volar cortices and occurs as a result of comminution or overlap of fragments; in these instances, simple angular correction will not restore to-

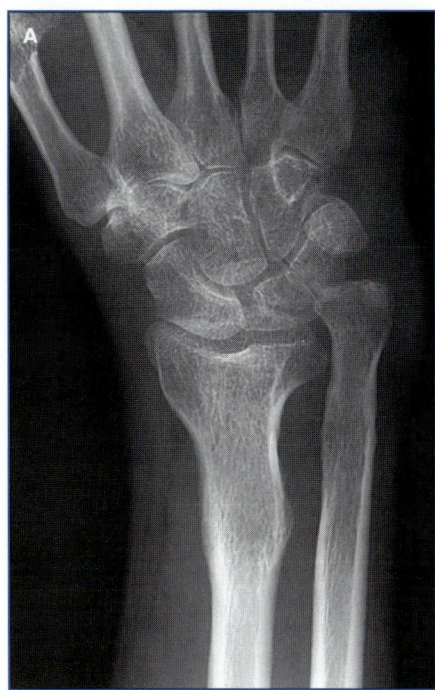
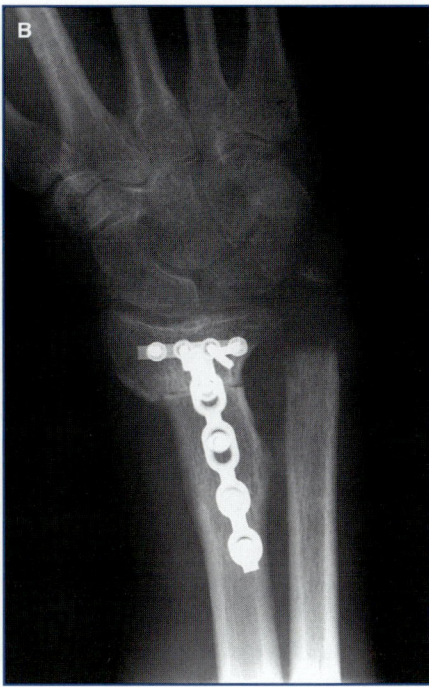

Figure 6 A 47-year-old man presents with constant ulnar-sided wrist pain 3 years after his second wrist fracture. The patient was considered low demand because of a concomitant head injury sustained at the time of the second fracture. **A,** PA view reveals almost 1 cm of ulnar positive variance and ulnar impaction. **B,** PA view after volar closing wedge osteotomy and Darrach resection.

tal radial length. In these more complex cases, an opening wedge osteotomy must be combined with a more extensive soft-tissue release and distraction of the entire epiphyseal fragment to restore the true length of the volar and dorsal cortices. In patients with more than 1 cm loss of real radial length, radial osteotomy alone is not likely to result in acceptable ulnar variance; therefore, adjunctive procedures to the distal ulna should be considered (**Figure 6**). In severe cases, correction of the deformity may not be possible, and a wrist arthrodesis must be considered (**Figure 7**).

Joint Incongruity

Assessment of the joint surfaces in a wrist malunion is critical but often difficult. Plain radiographs often are inaccurate.[13,14] Therefore, in a patient with a malunion and possible articular incongruity, CT with reconstruction should be obtained before corrective osteotomy is considered. Joint surface incongruity, as well as any associated osteoarthritis, may be the primary cause of pain and restricted motion after a malunion. Extra-articular corrective osteotomy of a typical dorsally tilted and shortened malunion is not likely to relieve symptoms in a patient with 2 mm or more of articular malalignment or early posttraumatic osteoarthritis.

However, joint-leveling osteotomy techniques for intra-articular malunions are rarely straightforward. The paucity of clinical results suggests that this complex procedure should be attempted only when the chance of success is high. Loss of fracture-line markings with progression of healing further increase the complexity; therefore, this surgery should be performed as soon as possible after the initial injury. The treatment of choice for an intra-articular malunion is prevention.

Rotational Deformity

As with all malunions, it is too simplistic to assume that deformity has occurred in only one plane. Recent studies have reported that many malunions have a rotational component in addition to angular deformity and shortening.[15] Although it often is believed that a supination deformity is associated with a dorsally tilted malunion, and a pronation deformity with

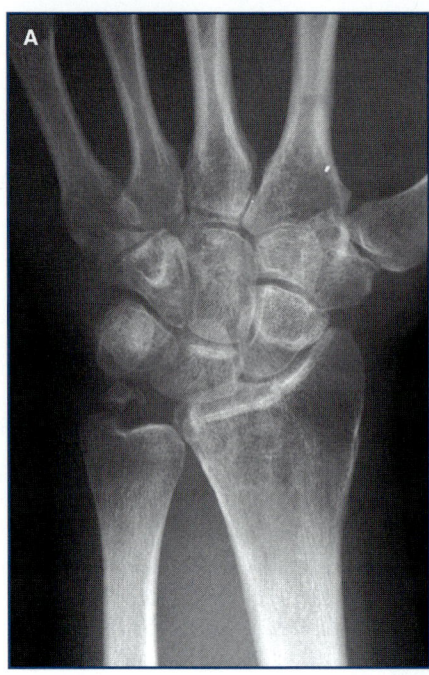
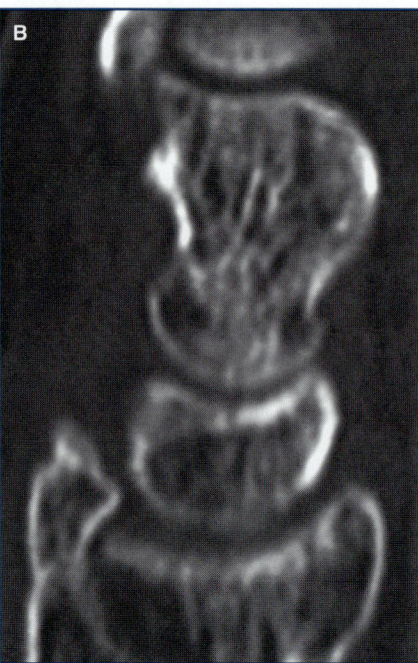

Figure 7 A 58-year-old man presents with persistent pain 1 year after a distal radius fracture. The treating physician told him that the fracture had healed nicely. **A,** PA view suggests an articular incongruity, but the cortical rim appears intact. **B,** CT scan reveals more than 2 mm of joint depression. Arthroscopy indicated that the joint surfaces were too damaged for intra-articular osteotomy to be considered.

a volarly tilted malunion, this relationship has not been consistently shown. In fact, the severity of the rotational malalignment does not appear to correlate with either malunion geometry or preoperative loss of forearm rotation. Use of radiographic and CT reconstruction techniques is proposed to better assess and correct rotational deformity. However, whether this correction is necessary is unclear because most studies report good outcomes after corrective osteotomy when rotational deformity has not been specifically corrected.[16-18]

Surgical Decision Making

Although all of the aforementioned radiographic parameters can be assessed fairly accurately, the decision to proceed with surgery must be made in proper context. An otherwise healthy, active 45-year-old patient and a low-demand resident of a nursing home have different thresholds for surgical intervention, even though they may have the same degree of radiographic malunion. The nature of the symptoms and physical findings, the patient's response to prior therapy, and the severity of the radiographic findings guide the decisions for proceeding with surgical treatment. Each patient's treatment must be individual-

ized, with significant attention paid to overall health and demands of any patient considering corrective osteotomy. Although severe deformity and/or compromised function lead to a fairly straightforward decision, caution must be exercised when considering surgery for patients with limited symptoms and poor past commitment to postsurgical therapy regimens. In younger patients, significant deformity but limited symptoms may constitute an excellent indication for surgery to prevent long-term problems. Finally, patients must be aware of the typical morbidities associated with surgery because hardware difficulties, postoperative infection, or bone graft complications can turn an otherwise minimally symptomatic malunion into a disaster.

Treatment

Surgical treatment for distal radius malunion generally can be grouped into one of two broad categories: reconstruction or salvage procedures. Reconstruction procedures, which restore the wrist anatomy to as normal as possible, typically entail a corrective osteotomy of the distal radius combined with a number of fixation and bone restoration options. Release of tight capsule or ligaments often compliments the osteotomy, and simultaneous ligamentous reconstruction of the unstable DRUJ and correction of a radial malunion have been described. Salvage procedures, generally indicated for severe deformity or osteoarthritis and in low-demand patients, are typically divided into two types of procedures: resections for functional improvement and arthrodeses for pain relief. In some complex situations, corrective procedures are combined with selected salvage procedures.

Reconstruction of Normal Anatomy

Candidates for reconstruction procedures are generally younger, active patients in search of pain relief and improved function. In general, these patients should be otherwise healthy and independent enough to participate in an outpatient hand therapy regimen or at least have sufficient resources and social support to ensure access to rehabilitation facilities. Furthermore, the condition of the surrounding soft tissues should be maximized; preoperative therapy to ensure maximal motion and strength can be helpful to prevent further setbacks during postoperative immobilization. Reconstruction for severe cosmetic and clinical deformity in older or ill individuals still may be reasonable, but in patients with decreased ability to attend rehabilitation sessions or comply with postoperative regimens, functional outcomes will be more limited.

Corrective osteotomy normally results in significant improvements in anatomic relationships, function, and symptoms in a properly selected patient.[16-18] Correction of the dorsal tilt to a neutral or slightly volarly tilted position is typical. Likewise, return of radial inclination and improvement in ulnar variance are predictably obtained. Wrist motion also is typically improved after corrective osteotomy, and grip strength typically improves to within 70% to 80% of the opposite, normal wrist. Cosmetic improvement from surgery is variable, with the most severe deformities demonstrating the most improvement.

Dorsal Radial Osteotomy

This workhorse operation has been described by many authors, and, therefore, many variations of the procedure exist. Preoperative planning combined with intraoperative identification of the osteotomy site are the keys to success of this procedure. Careful assessment of preoperative radiographs allows the surgeon to select the location of the osteotomy; in general, it should be performed as close as possible to the site of the prior fracture. However, it is prudent to make the osteotomy at least 15 to 20 mm proximal to the articular surface to ensure adequate distal bone for screw fixation. Although some surgeons believe formal preoperative templating is critical, we do not find it necessary given the advent of small intraoperative fluoroscopy units that allow for accurate intraoperative assessment of bony landmarks and the correction obtained. Clear understanding of the degree of shortening is required preoperatively.

In patients with mostly apparent shortening, ulnar variance will be restored to near normal with angular correction alone, whereas in patients with significant real shortening, a combination of soft-tissue releases and external fixation or a small-bone distractor is often required to restore adequate length. The soft-tissue releases include subperiosteal elevation of the second extensor compartment, the brachioradialis insertion, and the adjacent periosteum and adherent tissue radially until the entire base of the first extensor compartment is released. The entire base of the fourth and fifth compartments is released until the dorsal capsule of the DRUJ is exposed. We approach these releases in a stepwise fashion, working on both radial and ulnar sides until the distal fragment has been released sufficiently to allow adequate correction. A two-pin external fixator with a distraction device is sometimes helpful. The distal pin generally is inserted parallel to the radial artery surface to act as an alignment guide during distraction. Care must be taken to place pins away from the anticipated final position and to avoid pin cutout in the softer metaphyseal bone by moderating distraction force.

It often is helpful to drive one or two 1.6-mm Kirschner wires (K-wires) across the initial reduction to allow some temporary stabilization to better view the reduction on radiographs. This fixation is not rigid enough for healing but allows for temporary correction until the final hardware is placed.

Volar Radial Osteotomy

With a volarly tilted malunion, the surgical approach typically is from the volar surface. An incision through the flexor carpi radialis sheath, with reflection of the flexor pollicis longus and pronator quadratus to the ulnar side, provides full exposure of the volar aspect of the distal radius. The joint-marking technique and fluoroscopic guidance are similar to that for a dorsal radial osteotomy. The osteotomy is performed with care to ensure alignment of the osteotomy perpendicular to the long shaft of the radius and parallel with the joint surface. The last couple of millimeters of dorsal cortex should be penetrated with an osteotome. Protecting the soft tissues and avoiding penetration of the dorsal cortex with the saw are critical because of the intimate relationship of the extensor tendons against the radial and dorsal cortices. A complete carpal tunnel release generally is not performed at the time of surgery; however, in patients with severe deformity, transverse carpal ligament release may be prudent. This procedure increases the size of the volar incision but allows for more gentle retraction of the median nerve and flexor tendons.

Fixation of the Osteotomy

A wide variety of fixation choices for securing the osteotomy have been described. Traditionally, K-wires or Steinmann pins served as a mainstay for fixation. External fixation augmented by K-wires is used by some surgeons and is particularly time efficient if the fixator is already being used for distraction and length restoration. Currently, low-profile dorsal plates are the most practical and popular fixation option. All of these techniques generally are augmented with a piece of iliac crest graft that must be contoured to the defect before placement of final hardware.

Our preferred technique capitalizes on the development of precontoured fixed-angle plate technology. A stainless steel dorsal pi plate customized to fit the dorsal surface of the radius, or a hand-contoured, small-fragment locking T-plate, provides especially stable fixation because the screws and pins can be inserted into the distal fragment in a locking fashion. This blade plate equivalent generally obviates the need for a structural corticocancellous graft,[16] and we prefer simply packing morcellized cancellous graft into the defect. Although dorsal plates are the most popular fixation choice, extensor tendon irritation is a frequent problem. The intricate relationship of tendon and bone on the dorsal surface is disrupted by any dorsal plate, and as a result, secondary removal of plates for tendon irritation and prominence is common.

Bone Graft Choices

Historically, custom-fit corticocancellous bone grafts were the mainstay for osteotomies. Grafts generally were harvested from the iliac crest through standard oblique incision and contoured with rongeurs and bone cutters until the appropriate shape was obtained. Some surgeons even used foil or molded templates based on preoperative plans to help in graft construction. In conjunction with more stable dorsal plating options, some surgeons have moved toward packing cancellous graft into a rigidly stabilized dorsal defect, thereby simplifying the fitting and fixation portion of the procedure.[16] In most osteotomies where restoration of real length is limited to less than a few millimeters, cancellous grafts are especially safe. The revascularization and healing of the cancellous graft is rapid, with early healing often seen on radiographs at 5 or 6 weeks. Because of the secure internal fixation and rapid healing of the graft, gentle active motion can be initiated within 10 to 14 days after surgery, and all splinting can be discontinued by 8 weeks postoperatively.

Recent additions to current grafting technology have resulted in numerous substitutes for autogenous bone graft. Early reports on the use of some of these products in acute radius fractures have been promising; however, none has been rigorously tested in the setting of distal radius malunions. With time, and with combined experience in other body areas, some of these grafting substitutes may eventually replace autogenous graft harvests and their associated morbidity.

Complications

Careful assessment of intraoperative radiographs obtained by slightly tilting the PA and lateral views should virtually eliminate the possibility of hardware penetrating the joint. Plates placed dorsally on the radius are a frequent source of discomfort, even months after an osteotomy; therefore, patients should be advised before corrective surgery that plate removal may be necessary. Tendon irritation and tendinitis can lead to extensor tendon rupture; thus, close follow-up is necessary. Avoidance of titanium plates on the dorsal surface also may be advantageous because tendon adhesion with titanium is likely more problematic than with stainless steel. The recent addition of locked volar plate technology may reduce some of these hardware problems, but no clinical studies of these plates for malunion fixation currently exist. Impaired function of cutaneous nerves from retraction also is frequent after surgery, but most patients show improvement with time. While uncommon, infection can be a devastating problem requiring removal of hardware and graft.

Persistent pain at the iliac crest, cutaneous neuroma, pelvic fracture, and hematoma are well-recognized complications after bone graft harvest. Pain and neuroma usually can be minimized with the use of small incisions located at least 1 cm posterior to the anterior superior iliac spine. Likewise, limited soft-tissue stripping combined with trephination or trap-door approaches to the crest minimize devascularization and structural change at the crest itself. We find that the use of a coagulation-enhancing space occupier, such as a bioabsorbable gelatin sponge, in addition to a strong deep fascial closure, is helpful to reduce symptomatic hematoma formation. In certain individuals, harvesting from the distal femur or proximal tibia metaphyseal areas can help reduce complications.

Long-term complications include persistent loss of motion from capsular contracture and pain. DRUJ instability, pain, or stiffness and degeneration on the ulnar side of the wrist constitute some of the more difficult long-term problems. These latter issues are more fully addressed in the chapter on the DRUJ.

Salvage Procedures

In a selected group of low-demand or complex patients, the symptoms of a wrist malunion can be treated with alternate procedures that may be associated with less morbidity than opening wedge osteotomy and bone grafting. In some patients (minimal deformity or low demand), a simpler ulnar shortening procedure or excisional arthroplasty at the distal ulna may provide significant improvement in symptoms without the risk for complications of the more complex radial osteotomy.[19] Total wrist fusion represents the gold standard for treatment of persistent pain from joint derangement or osteoarthritis after radius malunion. Careful physical examination is required before this surgery is considered, however, and correlation with symptoms and radiographic or CT findings is key to identifying patients for whom this procedure will provide good resolution of symptoms. Limited radioscapholunate fusion may provide pain

relief and maintain some wrist motion for a subset of younger or high-demand patients with isolated radiocarpal arthritis. In the elderly or low-demand patient, total wrist arthroplasty after malunion has been described, but it has all of the associated risk and long-term complications typical of these somewhat experimental prostheses.

Prevention of Malunion

The most effective treatment for distal radius malunion is prevention. A combination of clinical and basic science studies have helped to define which fractures are predisposed to malunion after nonsurgical treatment.[1-5,7-10] A younger, active patient tends to be treated with a more aggressive surgical approach than a low-demand nursing home resident. However, with increasing life expectancy, many elderly patients remain active until late in life, and a poorly aligned distal radius malunion can be debilitating. Surgical treatment of fractures meeting the following criteria generally can prevent the development of late collapse or deformity. However, surgeon discretion is mandatory when applying these criteria to individual patients.

The first two criteria are dorsal tilting of the distal fragment beyond 20° and initial shortening of more than 5 mm on initial radiographs. These criteria imply increased metaphyseal comminution and, therefore, loss of bony support to any closed reduction obtained. Thus, fractures with these deformities generally require some form of surgical fixation to prevent late collapse.

The third criterion is articular displacement of greater than 1 to 2 mm. Given the paucity of reliable reconstruction options for intra-articular malunion and the real difficulty in truly assessing the magnitude of articular displacement, a low threshold for surgical treatment for articular injuries is advised. Open reduction can be especially complex in patients with high-energy injuries and extensive comminution. Opening a comminuted fracture only to be unable to reconstruct the numerous small articular fragments will result in an even worse outcome.

The fourth criterion is displaced shear-type fracture patterns (AO-ASIF type B injuries). These fractures require stabilization as a result of displacement of the carpal bones in association with the sheared fragments (**Figure 8**). Plate fixation is generally regarded as the treatment of choice for these fractures.

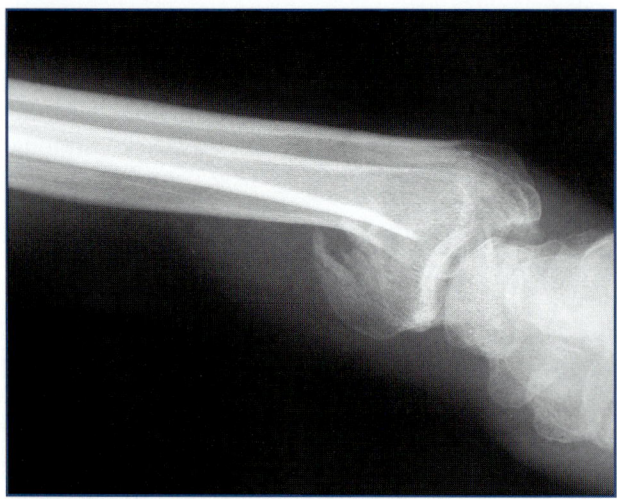

Figure 8 Lateral view of a displaced volar shear fracture that is not amenable to closed reduction and casting. A volar shift of the carpus in association with the volar radial fragment is identified. This fracture requires a volar buttress plate to secure the volar fragment and reduce the carpal bones.

The fifth criterion is fractures in young, active patients who sustain high-energy injuries. Fractures that result from falls from heights or high-speed crashes generally require surgical stabilization. These injuries are prone to instability, which is not surprising given the force required to fracture young, healthy bones.

An inadequate closed reduction also requires surgical treatment. Radiographic criteria of an inadequate reduction consist of failure to obtain volar tilt of 0° or more on the lateral view, persistent ulnar variance of more than 2 to 3 mm compared with the opposite normal wrist, and persistent articular surface displacement of more than 1 to 2 mm.

The last criterion involves fractures that redisplace on follow-up after closed reduction. Surgical reduction and fixation of fractures as late as 3 to 4 weeks after injury is generally less complex and associated with fewer morbidities than malunion surgery after complete healing. However, caution must be advised when treating fractures that present with loss of correction more than 3 to 4 weeks after injury. Disruption of early callus, softening of the metaphyseal bone, and loss of normal bony contours to align the fragments lead to significant difficulty in overcoming soft-tissue contracture, obtaining an accurate reduction,

and adequately fixing the fracture. In these patients, we find a generally more reliable strategy is to wait for solid bone healing, maximize outcome with early physical therapy, and advise corrective surgery 3 or more months after the injury.

MANAGEMENT AND OUTCOME SUMMARY

The patient in our case illustration has a typical history of a distal radius malunion. As in most of these cases, there were a number of missed opportunities to help prevent this outcome. On review of the initial injury radiographs, a number of markers of radiographic instability are present. The age of the patient (indicating young, healthy bone and, therefore, a high-energy fracture), dorsal tilting greater than 20°, and 5 mm of initial shortening all predict a high risk for malunion with nonsurgical treatment. The failure to obtain clear postreduction views to allow for correct radiographic assessment further contributed to a poor outcome. Finally, the advice to the patient that she would "do well" despite the obvious clinical and radiographic deformity denotes both a failure to appreciate the significant problems of distal radial malunions and a missed opportunity to communicate to the patient the difficulties she might experience from the malunion. Not surprisingly, this patient presented to a new surgeon with the typical multiple symptoms of a malunion—wrist pain, limited motion, cosmetic deformity, and carpal tunnel syndrome—and a strong resentment toward the physician who provided her initial treatment.

After a lengthy discussion with the patient about her current situation and the expected benefits and potential risks from corrective surgery, the patient elected to undergo a distal radial osteotomy. The need for an open carpal tunnel release also was discussed, and the patient elected for a release performed at the same time to prevent a possible second procedure and period of recovery. The surgery was done through a dorsal midline approach (**Figure 9, A**). The subcutaneous veins and sensory nerves were preserved or retracted, with communicating vessel branches or perforators cauterized as necessary. The extensor retinaculum was opened with a Z-shaped release, one limb based off of Lister's tubercle and the other based ulnarly (**Figure 9, B**). This release allows for reconstruction of retinaculum integrity on closure, when the bulk of a dorsal plate combined with restoration of length and angulation would typically prevent retinacular closure with a simple longitudinal release.

The base of the fourth compartment and the finger extensor tendons were then reflected subperiosteally to the ulnar side, and the extensor pollicis longus and the radial wrist extensors were retracted radially. The extensor pollicis longus was released from beneath the deep antebrachial fascia distal to the retinaculum to allow for more retraction. The extensor carpi radialis longus and brevis were reflected within the second compartment by subperiosteal elevation. This step provides wide exposure of the entire dorsal surface of the radius and allows easy access for release of the brachioradialis insertion onto the radial styloid. This latter maneuver may allow for improved restoration of length in patients with more problematic shortening. A segment of the posterior interosseous nerve at the base of the fourth compartment also can be resected at this time. This resection has some theoretical benefits for improved pain relief, but its utility has not been specifically examined in any clinical review of distal radial malunion corrections.

Although some authors recommend a capsulotomy to mark the distal articular surface, we find placement of a 1.6-mm K-wire under fluoroscopic control parallel to and just proximal to the articular surface less invasive (**Figure 9, C**). At the same time, the position of the osteotomy site in relation to the dorsal surface markings and the joint surface of the radius is marked (**Figure 9, D**). An oscillating saw with cooling saline irrigation was used to perform the osteotomy across the radial metaphysis with careful protection of the surrounding soft tissues. This cut was made parallel to the K-wire marking the radial articular surface, perpendicular to the long axis of the radius, and just proximal to the DRUJ. The saw is used to perform 90% of the cut across the bone, and a small osteotome is used to finish the cut across the last of the volar cortex to prevent damage to the pronator quadratus and tendons beyond.

The technique for distraction of the distal fragment is highly individualized. Some combination of manual distraction, laminar spreaders or self-retaining retractors, and external fixation is preferred by most authors. Placement of the K-wire parallel to the articular surface is a useful guide for restoring volar tilt, and is used in combination with fluoroscopy to confirm res-

toration of fairly normal radial angulation and volar tilt (**Figure 9, E**). In this patient, manual distraction with a small elevator and a bone pick was all that was required to obtain reduction. Restoration of volar tilt and ulnar variance was assessed after the reduction was temporarily secured with a second K-wire (**Figure 9, F**). The PA view of the opposite, normal wrist provides the comparison for the temporary reduction on the PA fluoroscopic view. In this patient, near neutral variance was obtained.

Next, we trimmed the plate to fit the distal fragment dorsal surface, removing a portion of Lister's tubercle to allow close contact with the bone. The plate was affixed to the distal fragment with two screws and then two locking pins. With the plate secured to the distal fragment, a final reduction of the distal fragment was performed under radiographic guidance and held in place while two screws were inserted into the proximal fragment (**Figure 9, G through I**). One of the advantages of this precontoured locking plate technique is that adjustments with the plate connected to the distal fragment in place are easy and allow for last-minute minor corrections of length or supination and pronation. The precontoured shape of the plate also ensures that with reduction of the plate onto the proximal fragment, near-normal angular anatomy will be restored. After a second radiographic check, the remaining proximal screw holes were filled.

Purely cancellous bone graft harvested from the iliac crest was then packed tightly into the defect (**Figure 9, J**). The retinaculum was closed in a lengthened position, the skin was closed, and dressings and a fiberglass sugar-tong splint were applied. A molded thermoplastic short arm splint was fabricated at the time of suture removal 12 days postoperatively. Gentle active and active-assist ROM was also initiated under the direction of a physical therapist at this time. After 6 weeks, radiographs revealed excellent incorporation of bone graft, and progressive physical therapy was instituted (**Figure 9, K and L**).

After 3 months, the patient was back to work and happy with the improved function. The carpal tunnel symptoms were completely resolved. She elected to terminate physical therapy at this time to focus on her work and as a result struggled with regaining full wrist motion. At 6-month follow-up, flexion had improved, but the patient felt limited by persistent pain and swelling over the radial styloid. Clinical examina-

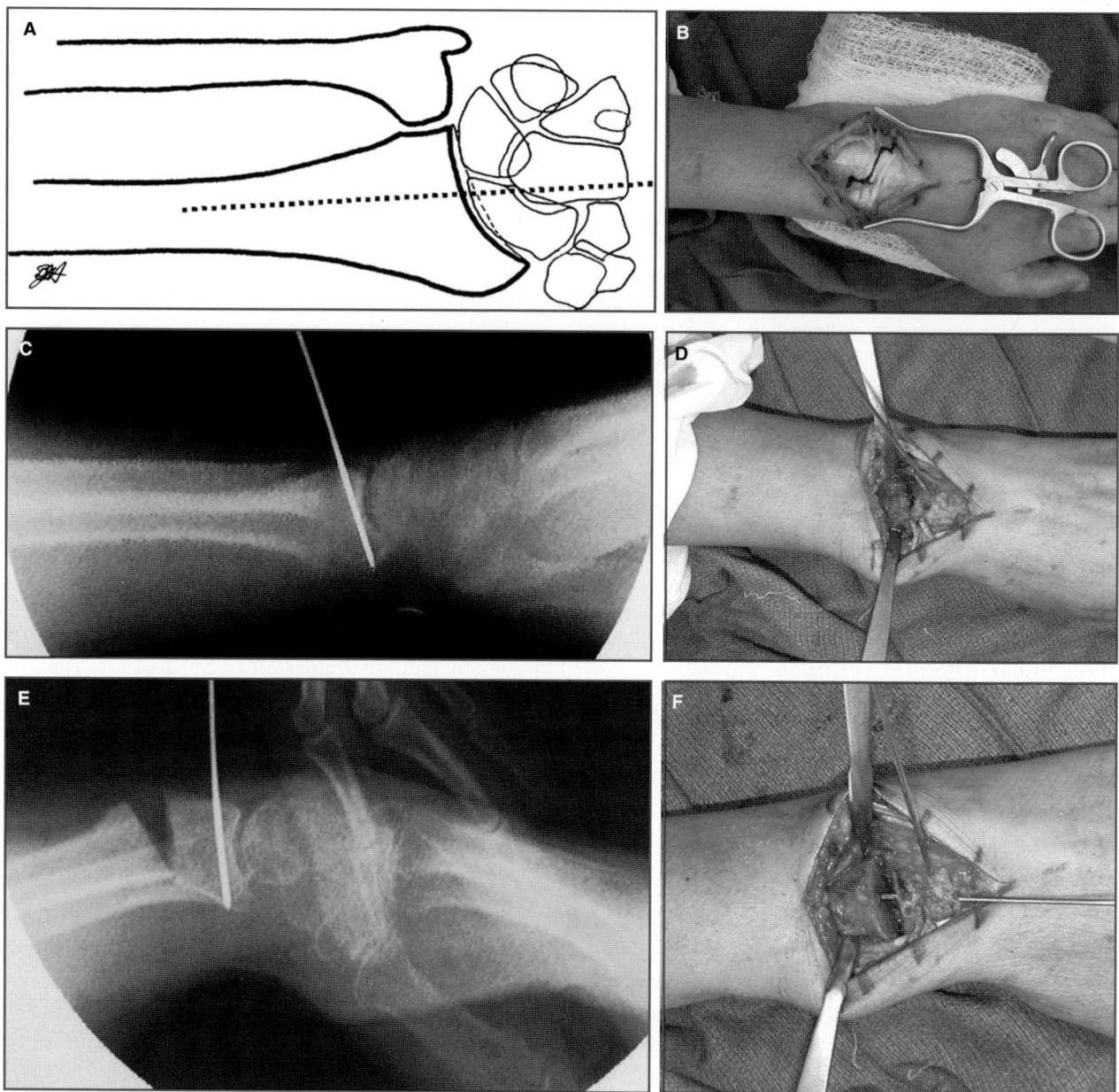

Figure 9 Surgical approach for dorsal corrective osteotomy. **A,** Alignment of skin incision. **B,** Intraoperative photograph showing retraction of subcutaneous tissues and Z-shaped release of extensor retinaculum. **C,** Intraoperative lateral radiograph identifies the location of a 1.6-mm K-wire to localize the articular surface. **D,** Intraoperative photograph showing the dorsal surface of the bone with a 1.6-mm K-wire marking the articular surface and the osteotomy site planned proximal to it. **E,** Intraoperative lateral radiograph identifying the articular surface after corrective manipulation. **F,** Intraoperative photograph showing correction temporarily secured with an additional 1.6-mm K-wire.

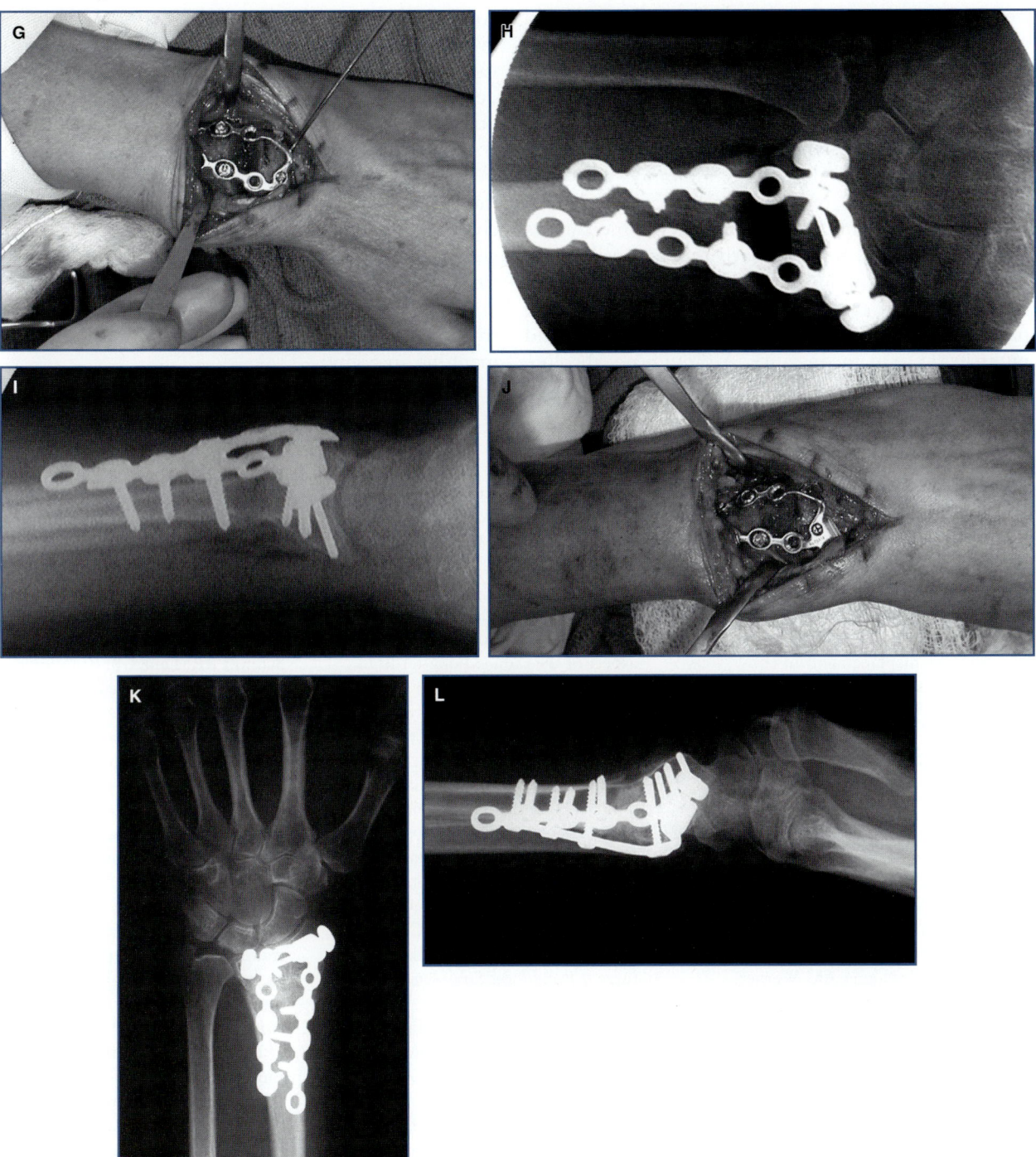

Figure 9 (continued)   **G,** The plate was affixed to the distal fragment and secured to the proximal fragment. PA **(H)** and lateral **(I)** views were obtained to check osteotomy alignment and hardware position. **J,** Final construct with cancellous bone graft tightly packed into the dorsal defect. PA **(K)** and lateral **(L)** radiographs obtained 5 weeks after surgery show that the alignment was maintained and early incorporation of bone graft. The patient was fitted for a removable splint and subsequently began physical therapy.

tion was consistent with irritation to the first and second extensor compartments, and all tendons were noted to be intact. At 10 months after the osteotomy, the plate was removed, and remaining symptoms resolved.

The assessment, planning, and execution of surgical treatment for distal radial malunion, as presented in this case example, represent a significant challenge. Although identifying the patient-specific indications for corrective osteotomy is clearly the responsibility of the surgeon, relative indications for surgical treatment of distal radial malunions include limited motion, pain, midcarpal instability, DRUJ dysfunction, and prearthritic joint incongruity. Although no absolute contraindications exist, limited functional disability, even in association with moderate deformity, constitutes a relative contraindication, especially in low-demand patients. By comparison, advanced degenerative changes limit the likely outcomes from corrective surgery. Finally, significant osteoporosis may represent a relative contraindication because of the difficulties in obtaining adequate fixation purchase after osteotomy. Although conduct of the surgery requires a careful assessment of preoperative deformity and knowledge of the various reconstructive and salvage options, the best results clearly result from precise restoration of the wrist's bony and ligamentous anatomy.

REFERENCES

1. Adams BD: Effects of radial deformity on distal radioulnar joint mechanics. *J Hand Surg [Am]* 1993;18:492-498.

2. Baratz ME, Des Jardins J, Anderson DD, Imbriglia JE: Displaced intra-articular fractures of the distal radius: The effect of fracture displacement on contact stresses in a cadaver model. *J Hand Surg [Am]* 1996;21:183-188.

3. Knirk JL, Jupiter JB: Intra-articular fractures of the distal end of the radius in young adults. *J Bone Joint Surg Am* 1986;68:647-659.

4. McQueen M, Caspers J: Colles fracture: Does the anatomical result affect the final function? *J Bone Joint Surg Br* 1988;70:649-651.

5. Short WH, Palmer AK, Werner FW, Murphy DJ: A biomechanical study of distal radial fractures. *J Hand Surg [Am]* 1987;12:529-534.

6. Taleisnik J, Watson HK: Midcarpal instability caused by malunited fractures of the distal radius. *J Hand Surg [Am]* 1984;9:350-357.

7. Trumble TE, Schmitt SR, Vedder NB: Factors affecting functional outcome of displaced intra-articular distal radius fractures. *J Hand Surg [Am]* 1994;19:325-340.

8. Aro HT, Koivunen T: Minor axial shortening of the radius affects outcome of Colles' fracture treatment. *J Hand Surg [Am]* 1991;16:392-398.

9. Catalano LW III, Cole RJ, Gelberman RH, et al: Displaced intra-articular fractures of the distal aspect of the radius: Long-term results in young adults after open reduction and internal fixation. *J Bone Joint Surg Am* 1997;79:1290-1302.

10. Kihara H, Palmer AK, Werner FW, Short WH, Fortino MD: The effect of dorsally angulated distal radius fractures on distal radioulnar joint congruency and forearm rotation. *J Hand Surg [Am]* 1996;21:40-47.

11. Jupiter JB, Fernandez DL: Complications following distal radial fractures. *J Bone Joint Surg Am* 2001;83:1244-1265.

12. Palmer AK, Werner FW: Biomechanics of the distal radioulnar joint. *Clin Orthop* 1984;187:26-35.

13. Cole RJ, Bindra RR, Evanoff BA, et al: Radiographic evaluation of osseous displacement following intra-articular fractures of the distal radius: Reliability of plain radiography versus computed tomography. *J Hand Surg [Am]* 1997;22:792-800.

14. Rozental TD, Bozentka DJ, Katz MA, Steinberg DR, Beredjiklian PK: Evaluation of the sigmoid notch with computed tomography following intra-articular distal radius fracture. *J Hand Surg [Am]* 2001;26:244-251.

15. Prommersberger KJ, Froehner SC, Schmitt RR, Lanz UB: Rotational deformity in malunited fractures of the distal radius. *J Hand Surg [Am]* 2004;29:110-115.

16. Ring D, Roberge C, Morgan T, Jupiter JB: Osteotomy for malunited fractures of the distal radius: A comparison of structural and nonstructural autogenous bone grafts. *J Hand Surg [Am]* 2002;27:216-222.

17. Fernandez DL: Correction of post-traumatic wrist deformity in adults by osteotomy, bone grafting and internal fixation. *J Bone Joint Surg Am* 1982;64:1164-1178.

18. af Ekenstam F, Hagert CG, Engkvist O, Tornvall AH, Wilbrand H: Corrective osteotomy of malunited fractures of the distal end of the radius. *Scand J Plast Reconstr Surg* 1985;19:175-187.

19. Tulipan DJ, Eaton RG, Eberhart RE: The Darrach procedure defended: Technique redefined and long-term follow-up. *J Hand Surg [Am]* 1991;16:438-444.

Chapter 2

NONUNION

Brian J. Harley, MD, FRCSC
Andrew K. Palmer, MD

CASE PRESENTATION

An otherwise healthy 37-year-old man presented to the emergency department with severe pain in the left wrist shortly after he tripped and fell down a flight of stairs. Examination revealed an obvious deformity to his left nondominant wrist but no open wounds. Radiographs revealed a comminuted distal radial fracture and a distal ulnar shaft fracture with extension of the fracture line into the radiocarpal joint surface (**Figure 1**). The fractures were treated acutely with open reduction and plate fixation of the distal ulnar shaft fracture and an adjustable spanning external fixator for the distal radial fracture (**Figure 2**).

The patient was discharged the following day and presented to the office 10 days postoperatively reporting moderately severe pain and marked swelling in the wrist, for which he has been taking oral analgesics every 4 hours. He denied having any neurologic abnormalities in his fingers. He was wearing a bulky dressing and a splint, and his arm was in a sling. Both were removed to reveal pin sites that appeared clean with slight serous drainage on the bandage. The ulnar-sided incision for the plate was healing well. Soft-tissue swelling was severe, and a few small fracture blisters were present, but circulation and sensation in his hand and fingers were normal. Range of motion (ROM) of the fingers was poor, limited both by swelling and pain. PA and lateral radiographs were obtained and revealed the distal ulnar shaft fracture to be in anatomic position and secured with a dynamic compression plate (**Figure 2**). The spanning external fixator was immobilizing the radial fracture in acceptable alignment.

The patient returned 1 week later reporting increasing pain at the pin sites, where there was erythema and drainage. Antibiotics were started, and the following week the pin sites improved, but finger ROM remained poor, and there still was moderate swelling. At 4 weeks, the tension in the fixator was released slightly. At 6 weeks postoperatively, the fracture appeared to be healing (**Figure 3**), but finger ROM continued to be poor. The fixator was removed after 7 weeks, he was fitted with a removable brace, and physical therapy was initiated. He returned 2 weeks after fixator removal and stated that he had made some progress at therapy. He reported persistent pain and swelling throughout the wrist. His strength was markedly reduced, and ROM was less than 30° in

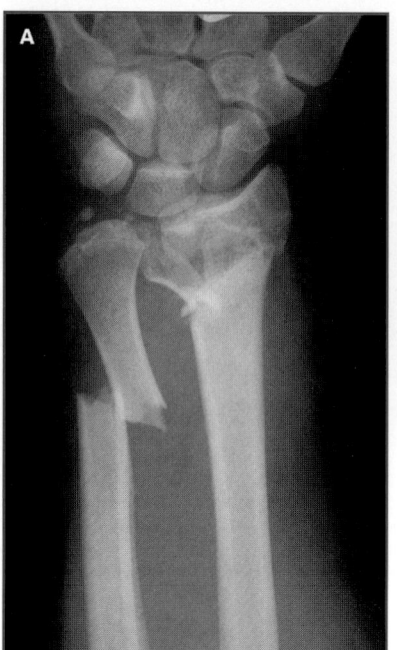

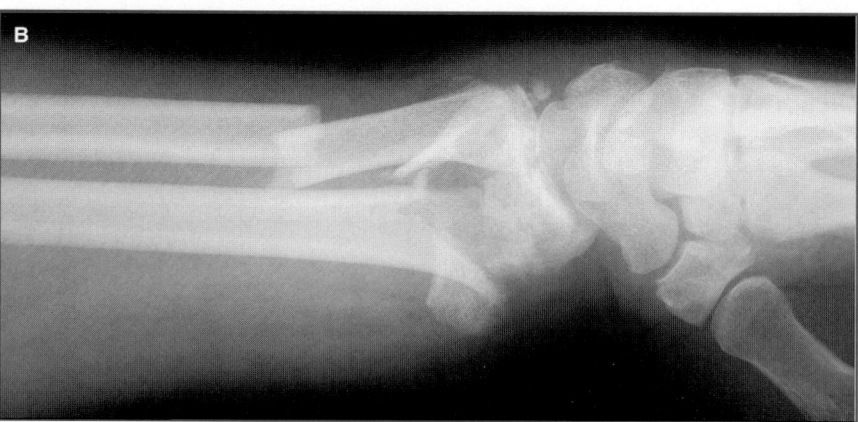

Figure 1 PA **(A)** and lateral **(B)** radiographs show a comminuted intra-articular distal radius fracture in conjunction with a distal ulnar diaphyseal fracture.

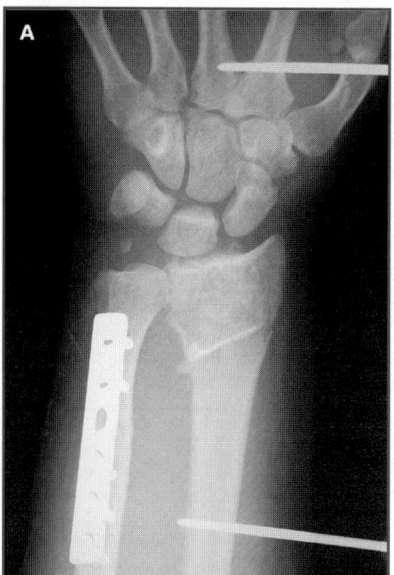

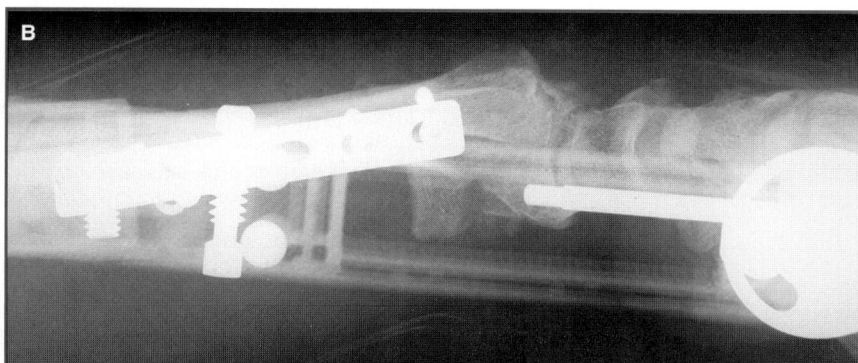

Figure 2 PA **(A)** and lateral **(B)** views of the fracture after open reduction and plate fixation of the ulnar shaft fracture and external fixation of the distal radius fracture. Ulnar alignment is anatomic, and the radiocarpal articular surface, radial length, and radial inclination have been restored on the PA view. Metaphyseal comminution is marked. The lateral view reveals acceptable radial alignment but with a displaced and rotated volar cortical fragment.

both flexion and extension. He had point tenderness to palpation of a more prominent ulnar head and a slight increase in distal radioulnar joint (DRUJ) mobility compared with the opposite wrist.

The PA radiograph revealed a marked loss of radial length with a resultant increase in ulnar variance, and the metaphyseal fracture line remained clearly visible, although some early callus was now evident at the margins (**Figure 4**). There has been a clear loss of the initial reduction and a resultant increase in the volar tilt of the radius. Dorsal subluxation of the distal ulna was now evident on the lateral view. A small ulnar

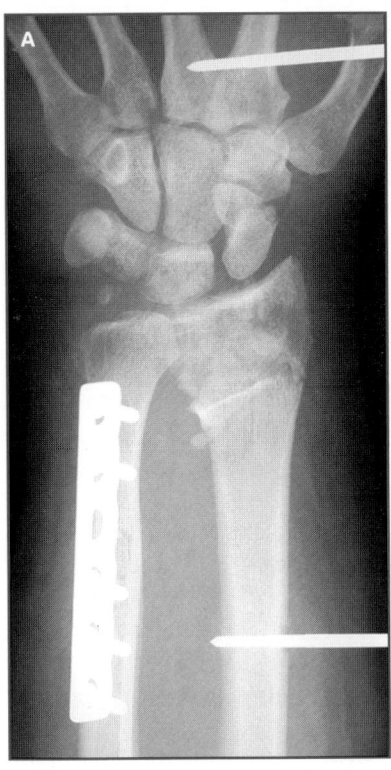

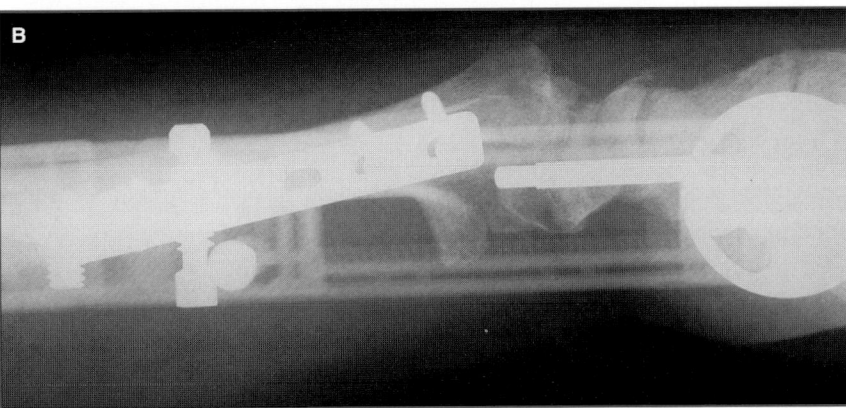

Figure 3 PA **(A)** and lateral **(B)** radiographs after 6 weeks in an external fixator. The fracture lines are becoming more indistinct, and plans were made to remove the fixator.

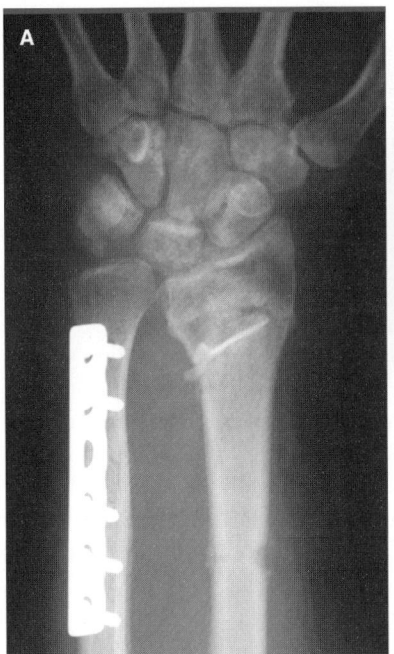

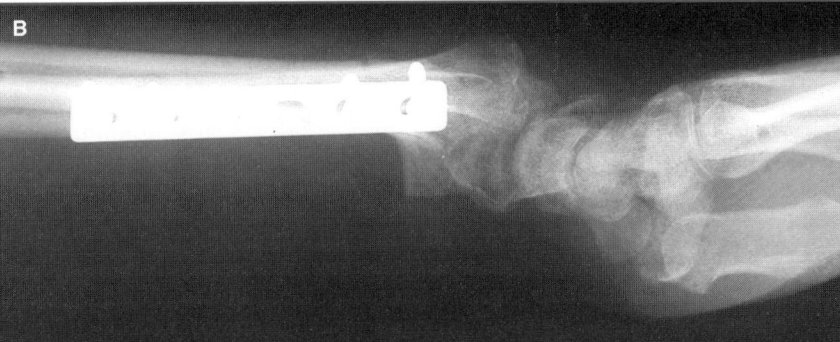

Figure 4 PA **(A)** and lateral **(B)** radiographs 4 weeks after fixator removal. The PA view reveals marked loss of radial length, a distinct metaphyseal fracture line, and poor callus formation. The lateral view reveals 25° of volar tilt and increased palmar displacement of the epiphyseal fragment.

styloid fragment had not united, but the carpal alignment appeared normal.

DISCUSSION

Despite the administration of what is believed to be adequate treatment, some fractures heal too slowly or simply fail to heal. A nonunion is defined as a failure of progression of bone healing, whereas a delayed union occurs when healing progresses significantly more slowly than expected, such that reduction is lost and/or surgical intervention generally is indicated. Although there is no obvious cause for some fracture nonunions, most occur as a result of one or more typical fracture variables. Patient-specific factors, such as open or high-energy fractures, deep infection, pathologic fractures, poor local blood supply, systemic disease, or malnutrition, can contribute to poor healing. Treatment-related factors, such as extensive soft-tissue stripping, insufficient immobilization, and excessive distraction across the fracture site with a resultant gap, also can contribute to nonunions. Attention to these latter factors is typically sufficient to prevent development of nonunions at the distal radius, but when they do occur, radial nonunion is troublesome and generally requires a prolonged treatment course. By comparison, nonunions at the distal ulna are common after wrist fracture and of variable significance. Each site is, therefore, described separately.

Radial Metaphysis

The development of nonunion after a wrist fracture is not an acceptable outcome; therefore, management focuses on restoring normal skeletal alignment, often with surgical correction. However, as the frequency of surgical interventions for these acute fractures has increased, so too has the realization that delayed or impaired healing at the radial metaphysis can occur. Nonunion at this well-vascularized site of metaphyseal bone is uncommon, but several authors have reported on delayed union or nonunion of the distal radius.[1-5] Although the causes for nonunion are variable, the combination of the following factors is most likely at the root of the problem: (1) surgical intervention to restore radial length, often with a resultant bone gap; (2) an ulnar shaft or neck fracture in conjunction with the distal radial fracture; (3) an inadequate stabilization method; and (4) an inadequate duration of immobilization. In our experience, patients with a high-energy mechanism of injury, generally with severe associated soft-tissue injuries, also have an increased risk of delayed union or nonunion.

Clinical Assessment

Patients with nonunions or delayed unions typically report persistent pain and/or progressive deformity at presentation. Often they have failed to improve during the first few weeks of physical therapy or have been unable to complete physical therapy because of pain. The pain is localized to the area of the fracture, and persistent swelling is typical. If the external fixator or pins have been removed, pain and motion at the fracture site may be perceived with manipulation. If the initial injury was treated with internal fixation, pain and motion at the fracture site generally are not present unless loosening or failure of the hardware has occurred.

Infection should always be considered, although it is uncommon in this well-vascularized area. A fluctuant area or drainage from the fracture site or surgical incisions will raise clinical suspicion of infection. A C-reactive protein, erythrocyte sedimentation rate, and complete blood count with a differential may provide some helpful information, but a negative screen does not rule out a low-grade infection. Cultures of the nonunion site are the only way to accurately diagnose infection in the usual patient.

Radiographic Assessment

Patients with a distal radius metaphyseal fracture should show obvious progress toward healing within 3 months of fracture; those with limited to no healing by 4 months can be considered to have a nonunion. Radiographs should be carefully scrutinized to identify subtle changes in radial inclination or volar tilt because motion of the fragments after immobilization is discontinued is pathognomonic for a nonunion. True PA and lateral radiographs must be obtained, however, because oblique views can impair accurate assessment of radiographic features.

Treatment

Selecting the proper course of treatment for a patient who has persistent pain at only 2 or 3 months after the fracture, often after removal of an external fixator, with slow progression toward complete healing is clearly difficult. If fracture alignment remains acceptable, then continued immobilization and close observation for an additional 4 to 6 weeks may be indicated. Smoking cessation, nutritional counseling, and some gentle physical therapy to promote motion of the adjacent joints and reduce swelling may improve healing potential and reduce symptoms. An additional period of casting, however, can further prolong the period of disability and ultimately make alignment worse; thus, careful follow-up is mandatory. Addition of one of a variety of external bone growth stimulators may promote healing, and anecdotal cases have been reported. However, definitive evidence of a clinical advantage is lacking, and we have no personal experience with these modalities. A patient with unacceptable alignment generally can be counseled on the advantages of surgical realignment and fixation to correct both fragment position and delayed healing. Nonsurgical treatment for persistent nonunion after 4 months is indicated only for patients with limited functional demands.

Surgical treatment for this condition is similar to that for distal radius malunion. Open correction of the malalignment with stabilizing internal fixation and bone grafting to fill the resultant defect is advised. Surgical restoration of bony anatomy typically improves radiocarpal and radioulnar alignment and generally improves DRUJ stability. If secure internal fixation is obtained, an early physical therapy program can be instituted. With solid union, a passive stretching program and an aggressive rehabilitation program are instituted. Restoration of ROM and strength generally results in a satisfied patient. Given the prolonged initial period of immobilization followed by a second surgical intervention and period of immobilization, patients must be counseled to expect permanent loss of some strength and motion.

Differentiation between atrophic and hypertrophic nonunions at the level of the radial metaphysis has not been reported, likely because of the low overall incidence of this condition. In our experience, distal radial nonunions tend to show characteristics more indicative of an atrophic nonunion; therefore, we prefer to use autologous bone graft in all patients. We also perform meticulous débridement of fibrous tissue at the site of the nonunion and restoration of the medullary canal of the proximal fragment. Although use of bone graft substitutes to fill bone void in the acute fracture setting is gaining popularity, the efficacy of these alternatives in the nonunion setting has not been documented.

In rare instances, restoring wrist architecture simply is not feasible. Caution must be exercised when attempting to achieve healing of distal fragments that are so small they are unamenable to fixation. Nonunions with marked displacement of the distal fragment or increased ulnar variance usually are associated with severe soft-tissue contractures that can prevent adequate realignment. Infected nonunions also represent a challenging situation and after a thorough débridement may preclude reconstruction. For these complex scenarios, as well as in most patients with one or more prior failed attempts at union, total wrist arthrodesis is the treatment of choice.

As with all cases of abnormal healing at the wrist, the best treatment of radial metaphysis nonunion is prevention. Close observation of fracture healing is important in all cases, but in patients who have had internal fixation, scrutinizing all postoperative radiographs for signs of hardware back out or loosening can help identify signs of impending nonunion that require treatment. When spanning external fixators are used for fracture fixation, excessive distraction must be avoided. Although no specific guidelines exist, we prefer to augment fixators with pins and liberally insert allograft or commercial bone graft substitutes into areas of significant metaphyseal comminution to increase fracture stability, improve healing, and reduce the duration of fixation.[6]

Ulnar Styloid

The ulnar styloid is easily identified on radiographs as the prominence at the distal end of the ulnar head. Various shapes and sizes exist, but the actual functional importance of this bony protuberance is uncertain. What is clear, however, is its relationship to the critical surrounding soft tissues. The triangular fibrocartilage complex (TFCC) originates from the base of the styloid, and the ulnar collateral complex, volar ulnocarpal ligaments, and subsheath of the extensor carpi ulnaris (ECU) have intimate relationships with the more distal aspects of the styloid.[7] Although the distal bony portion of the styloid generally may be discarded, maintaining the soft-tissue sleeve around the styloid plays a key role in DRUJ stability.

Unlike nonunion of the distal radial metaphysis, ulnar styloid nonunion is a common outcome of wrist fractures. This nonunion likely occurs because small fracture fragments and extensive soft-tissue attachments to the styloid preclude secure immobilization with routine nonsurgical treatment. In a typical population of patients with wrist fractures, ulnar styloid fractures are identified in up to 75% of patients; yet despite attention to restoring angular alignment and the length parameters of the distal radius, radiographic nonunion of the ulnar styloid occurs in almost half of these styloid fractures.[8-10] Although surgical intervention of displaced unstable distal radius fractures has become common, surgical management of fractures of the ulnar styloid is not and generally is limited to those injuries in which there is DRUJ instability.

Prevention of Nonunion

As with most scenarios in which poor healing can result in increased morbidity, prevention of nonunion is clearly advantageous. Unfortunately, there is no universally accepted set of indications for surgical treatment of ulnar styloid fractures. Surgical fixation of all ulnar styloid fractures is clearly overly aggressive, given the low rate of symptomatic ulnar styloid nonunions in a typical wrist fracture population.[11] With the evolution of clearer indications for surgical fixation of the styloid and improvements in the available implants, many symptomatic ulnar styloid nonunions can be prevented. We typically tend to treat most styloid fractures nonsurgically with the following two exceptions: First, any styloid fracture associated with moderate to severe DRUJ instability or a dislocation is repaired. If the styloid fragment is too small, it is excised and the TFCC repaired back to bone. Second, a large ulnar styloid fragment that extends into the foveal base is significantly easier to treat acutely (generally at the time of distal radius fixation) than when a nonunion develops, both in terms of

fragment reduction and fixation. Furthermore, it is predisposed to DRUJ instability in the long term.[12]

Clinical Assessment

The actual incidence of symptomatic ulnar styloid nonunion is not clearly reported in the literature. Early studies by Knirk and Jupiter[8] focused attention on the increased rate of adverse outcomes in patients with radiographic styloid nonunion. The large body of evidence collected following this study presents contrasting results, however, with many authors concluding that styloid nonunion did not account for poorer functional results.[13-15] Unfortunately, most authors reporting complications do not clearly describe whether the symptoms are the result of low-grade instability, associated TFCC tears, or the styloid nonunion itself.

The key to selecting the proper treatment strategy seems to be determining whether a patient's symptoms result from DRUJ instability, irritation at the nonunion site, or a combination of both. Therefore, when examining patients with ulnar-sided pain and disability after a wrist fracture, it is important to distinguish pain at the nonunion site from any instability on stress testing of the DRUJ. For this test, the examiner stabilizes the radial metaphysis between thumb and index finger of one hand while shucking the distal ulnar shaft in a dorsal and volar direction with the other hand. Testing generally should be performed in both pronation and supination, and comparing the affected wrist with the opposite, normal wrist is required to determine whether the laxity on the affected side is consistent with the patient's natural laxity at the DRUJ.

Treatment

Hauck and associates[16] classified symptomatic ulnar styloid nonunions as either one of two types: those with a stable DRUJ (type I) and those with an unstable DRUJ (type II). Although this dichotomy seems rather arbitrary given the spectrum of instability obtained from a clinical examination, the concept is important. If a patient presents with ulnar-sided pain and a stable DRUJ, simple subperiosteal excision of the styloid fragment can provide excellent symptom relief and prevent long-term degeneration of the ECU tendon. In general, these patients tend to have smaller, more distally located styloid nonunions.

However, in a patient with symptoms localized to the styloid nonunion and increased DRUJ instability compared with the opposite wrist, maintaining ulnar-sided soft-tissue structures during surgery is vital. If the nonunion fragment is comminuted or too small for implant fixation, then excision of the bone fragments with reattachment of the TFCC and surrounding capsule to the remaining ulna is indicated. This procedure is easily accomplished through an ulnar-sided approach, with care taken to protect the dorsal cutaneous branch of the ulnar nerve. A real advantage of this approach is the visualization of the base of the styloid and fovea with minimal disruption of the remaining ECU subsheath. Pulling nonabsorbable sutures through bone tunnels, or using suture anchors, can allow for excellent restoration of the ulnar soft-tissue sleeve. The DRUJ is pinned in neutral rotation just proximal to the joint for 4 to 6 weeks only for patients with marked instability or for patients who may be noncompliant with a postoperative period of forearm immobilization.

If a large styloid fragment is not united at the base, surgical preparation of the nonunion site followed by rigid internal fixation (and bone grafting if necessary) is straightforward and reliable, though more challenging than acute fracture fixation (**Figure 5**). We prefer a direct ulnar-sided approach for this technique and use a fluoroscope to ensure hardware placement is adequate. Although Kirschner wires (K-wires) and a tension band have been used extensively, many patients describe irritation from the hardware and request removal.[16] We therefore prefer the use of a headless screw, which can be buried within the styloid. The smallest implant diameters available in these screws are required, and a length of 18 to 24 mm is generally adequate to span the nonunion and obtain acceptable purchase in proximal and distal fragments. Care must be exercised to avoid fragmenting the styloid; therefore, the screw cannot be used in a small styloid. The absence of clear anatomic landmarks to guide fragment reduction and rotational alignment and the careful soft-tissue dissection required to mobilize the fragment contribute to the increased complexity of this procedure. Bone gaps or small voids in the medial cortex are frequently seen, and addition of cancellous graft from the distal radius may be required.

MANAGEMENT AND OUTCOME SUMMARY

This patient has a history typical of a nonunion of a distal radius fracture. A number of predictors for the nonunion occurred and, while clearer in hindsight, a number of opportunities to help prevent this outcome were missed. The age of the patient and the energy of the fracture, as evident by the mechanism of injury and the marked swelling at presentation, were nonunion risk factors. The associated distal ulnar shaft fracture was a further predictor of nonunion. Most predictive, however, was the external fixation technique used for fracture immobilization. The distraction at the radiocarpal joint suggests overdistraction, and despite attempts to modify the reduction with fixator adjustments in the postoperative period, an anatomic reduction could not be obtained. Comminution in the metaphyseal region was marked and a large volar cortical fragment rotated out of alignment. Neither augmentation pins nor bone graft was used in an attempt to correct the lost radial inclination, fill the metaphyseal defect, or further stabilize the fracture. Not surprisingly, when the external fixator was removed at 7 weeks, the radial fracture collapsed, and the patient presented with the typical constellation of multiple symptoms of a nonunion: wrist pain and swelling, limited and painful motion, and increased clinical and radiographic deformity.

After a discussion of the expected benefits from surgical realignment, fixation, and bone grafting, and of the possible risks of surgery compared to continued nonsurgical treatment, the patient elected for surgical repair. The surgical approach was volar, using the interval between the flexor carpi radialis and the radial artery to expose the deep muscle compartments. The pronator and the flexor pollicis longus were elevated from the volar surface of the radius, and a small amount of soft callus was identified at the site of the prior fracture. This callus was easily displaced from the bone, and the nonunion site was exposed. The brachioradialis was released from the radial styloid fragment to allow for fragment distraction.

A small, wide osteotome was used to cut through some bridging bone on the radial metaphysis and then used to manipulate the fragment back into correct

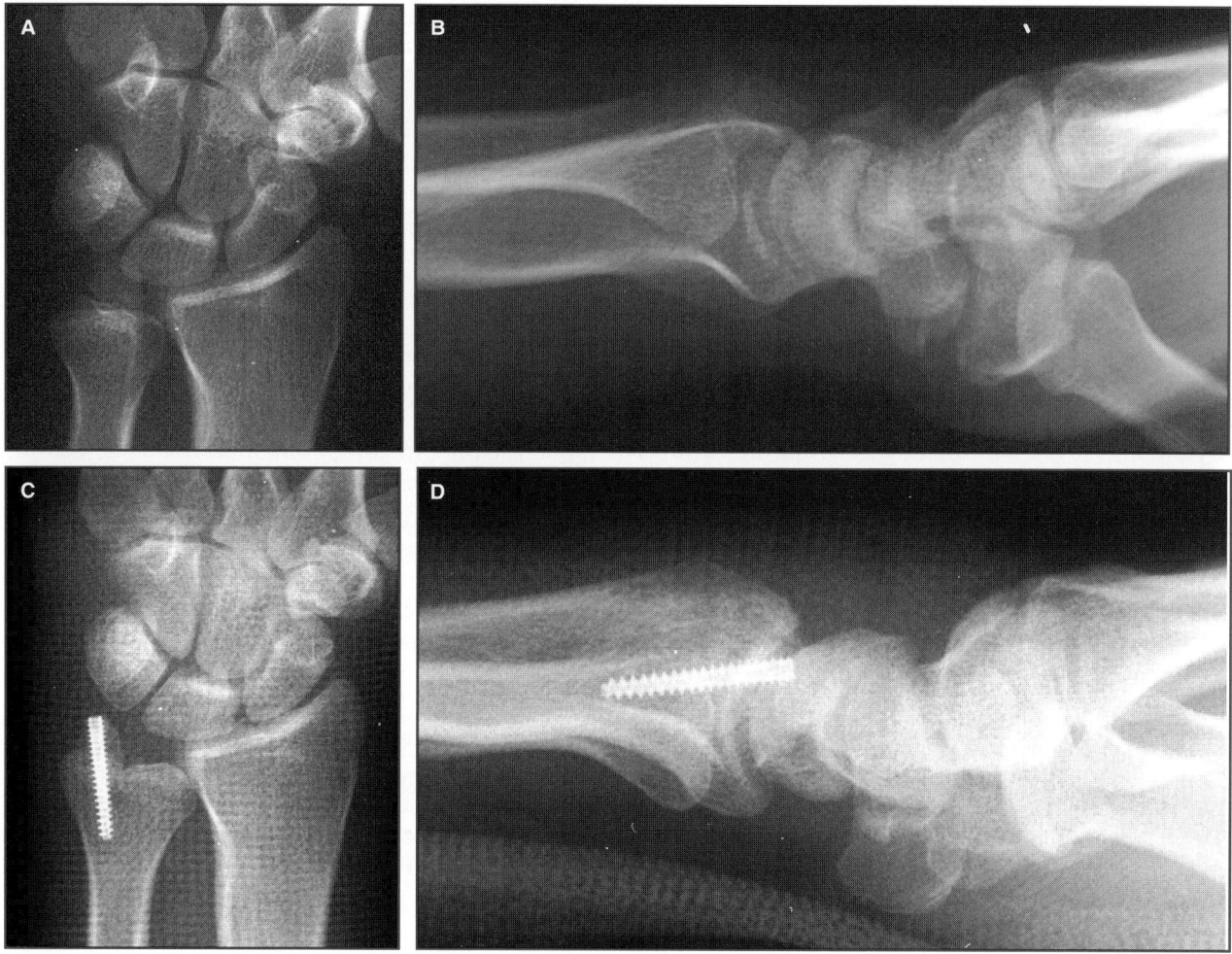

Figure 5 A 28-year-old man presented with ulnar-sided wrist pain 2 years after a wrist fracture that was treated with closed reduction and casting. **A,** The PA view reveals mild radial deformity and a hypertrophic ulnar styloid. **B,** The lateral view reveals the large ulnar styloid nonunion and acceptable radial and DRUJ alignment. PA **(C)** and lateral **(D)** views after open reduction and grafting with insertion of a headless compression screw.

alignment. The nonunion site was completely débrided of fibrous tissue with the use of small curets and rongeurs, and the fracture edges were decorticated with a small, narrow osteotome. A volar plate was contoured to the volar surface and secured to both proximal and distal fragments (**Figure 6**). Bone graft harvested from the iliac crest was then packed in the remaining defect. Dressings and a sugar-tong splint were applied after final wound closure.

Postoperatively, the patient was treated in a cast for 6 weeks, and physical therapy was initiated on cast

removal. The patient experienced rapid improvement in wrist function in the first 2 months postoperatively and discontinued his brace against medical advice. Complete radiographic union proceeded unimpeded, but clinically the patient plateaued at 6 months postoperatively with only 55° of wrist flexion, and 50° of wrist extension. He was pain free at rest but reported aching with prolonged use, and his grip strength improved to only 80% of his opposite extremity. Examination of his DRUJ revealed subtle instability in pronation compared with his opposite wrist.

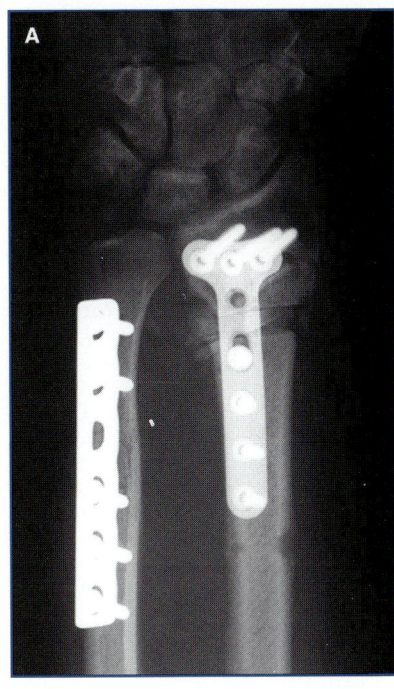

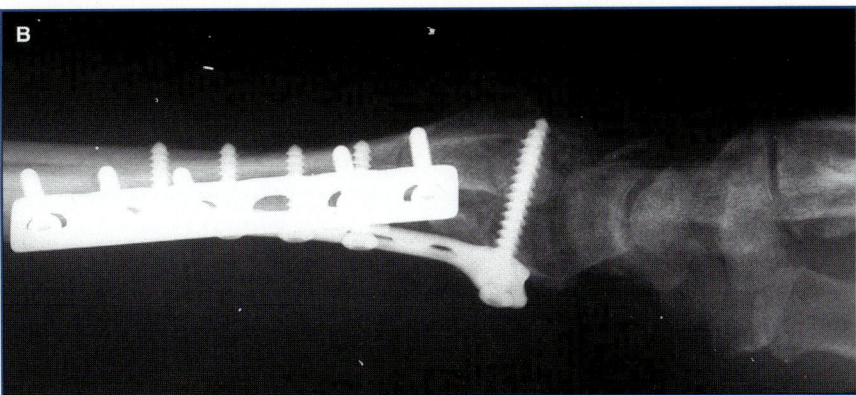

Figure 6 PA **(A)** and lateral **(B)** radiographs after open reduction and iliac crest bone grafting with volar plate fixation of a distal radius nonunion. Radial length and inclination have been restored.

Radial nonunion after wrist fracture is uncommon. But as evident in this case, nonunion often can be predicted by certain fracture and fixation variables. Following standard techniques for treatment of these fractures and avoiding overdistraction with an external fixator can help avoid this problem. When a nonunion is identified, rigid fixation and bone grafting to restore anatomy and stability is the treatment of choice.

Ulnar styloid nonunions, by comparison, are common. Most are asymptomatic and simply can be observed. To prevent symptomatic nonunions, internal fixation for large and/or unstable styloid fragments at the time of acute injury is recommended. However, simple excision of small fragments with repair of the soft-tissue sleeve or fixation and grafting of large styloid fragments is indicated for symptomatic nonunions.

REFERENCES

1. Fernandez DL, Ring D, Jupiter JB: Surgical management of delayed union and nonunion of distal radius fractures. *J Hand Surg [Am]* 2001;26:201-209.
2. McKee MD, Waddell JP, Yoo D, Richards RR: Nonunion of distal radial fractures associated with distal ulnar shaft fractures: A report of four cases. *J Orthop Trauma* 1997;11:49-53.
3. Segalman KA, Clark GL: Un-united fractures of the distal radius: A report of twelve cases. *J Hand Surg [Am]* 1998;23:914-919.
4. Smith VA, Wright TW: Nonunion of the distal radius. *J Hand Surg [Br]* 1999;24:601-603.
5. Weber SC, Szabo RM: Severely comminuted distal radial fractures as an unsolved problem: Complications associated with external fixation and pins and plaster techniques. *J Hand Surg [Am]* 1986;11:157-165.
6. Leung KS, Shen WY, Leung PC, et al: Ligamentotaxis and bone grafting for comminuted fractures of the distal radius. *J Bone Joint Surg Br* 1989;71:838-842.
7. Ishii S, Palmer AK, Werner FW, Short WH, Fortino MD: An anatomic study of the ligamentous structure of the triangular fibrocartilage complex. *J Hand Surg [Am]* 1998;23:977-985.
8. Knirk JL, Jupiter JB: Intra-articular fractures of the distal end of the radius in young adults. *J Bone Joint Surg Am* 1986;68:647-659.
9. Richards RS, Bennett JD, Roth JH, Milne K Jr: Arthroscopic diagnosis of intra-articular soft tissue injuries associated with distal radial fractures. *J Hand Surg [Am]* 1997;22:772-776.

10. Villar RN, Marsh D, Rushton N, Greatorex RA: Three years after Colles' fracture: A prospective review. *J Bone Joint Surg Br* 1987; 69:635-638.

11. Sennwald GR, Della Sanata D: Unstable distal radial fractures treated by external fixation: An analytical review. *Scand J Plast Reconstr Surg Hand Surg* 2002;36: 226-230.

12. May MM, Lawton JN, Blazar PE: Ulnar styloid fractures associated with distal radius fractures: Incidence and implications for distal radioulnar joint instability. *J Hand Surg [Am]* 2002;27:965-971.

13. Catalano LW III, Cole RJ, Gelberman RH, et al: Displaced intra-articular fractures of the distal aspect of the radius: Long-term results in young adults after open reduction and internal fixation. *J Bone Joint Surg Am* 1997;79: 1290-1302.

14. Roysam GS: The distal radio-ulnar joint in Colles' fractures. *J Bone Joint Surg Br* 1993;75:58-60.

15. Oskarsson GV, Aaser P, Hjall A: Do we underestimate the predictive value of the ulnar styloid affection in Colles' fractures? *Arch Orthop Trauma Surg* 1997; 116:341-344.

16. Hauck RM, Skahen J III, Palmer AK: Classification and treatment of ulnar styloid nonunion. *J Hand Surg [Am]* 1996;21:418-422.

Chapter 3

The Distal Radioulnar Joint

Brian J. Harley, MD, FRCSC
Andrew K. Palmer, MD

Case Presentation

A 28-year-old man who presents with pain and decreased strength in his left wrist and hand states that he broke his wrist almost 8 years ago while serving in the military and was treated with a cast at that time. The fracture healed, but he has had persistent ulnar-sided pain ever since the cast was removed. The pain is becoming worse, and he believes that his grip strength is becoming weaker. He notes that with rotational movements of the wrist he has a painful clicking on the ulnar side that has been causing him to drop objects at times. He describes intermittent bracing of his affected wrist with the opposite hand to "put it back into place." He has quit his job as a warehouse manager because he can no longer lift heavy objects. He is otherwise healthy and denies any other joint symptoms.

Examination reveals minimal swelling on the ulnar aspect of the wrist, but the ulnar head is prominent compared with the opposite wrist. He reports tenderness to palpation of the ulnar aspect of the wrist, both volarly and dorsally, although he poorly localizes the site of maximal tenderness. Range of motion is reduced in all directions compared with the opposite wrist, and passive ulnar deviation causes him to withdraw the hand in pain. Pronation and supination are full, but painful. On stress testing of the distal radioulnar joint (DRUJ), gross subluxation of the distal ulna with no obvious end points is identified. The ulna is unstable in both dorsal and palmar directions in all positions of forearm rotation, especially pronation. The opposite wrist is tight on stressing of the DRUJ in both pronation and supination.

A PA view of the affected wrist reveals normal inclination of the distal radius but markedly increased positive ulnar variance compared with the unaffected wrist (**Figure 1**, *A* and *B*). Several small ossicles are visualized at the distal aspect of the ulnar styloid. The lateral view of the affected wrist reveals normal radial anatomy and a reduced ulnar head (**Figure 1**, *C*). Views of the left elbow reveal an intact radial head and neck, and the joint appears normal (**Figure 1**, *D*).

Discussion

Ulnar-sided pain and/or instability after a fracture of the distal radius is a common occurrence. Although advances in technology over the past 25 years

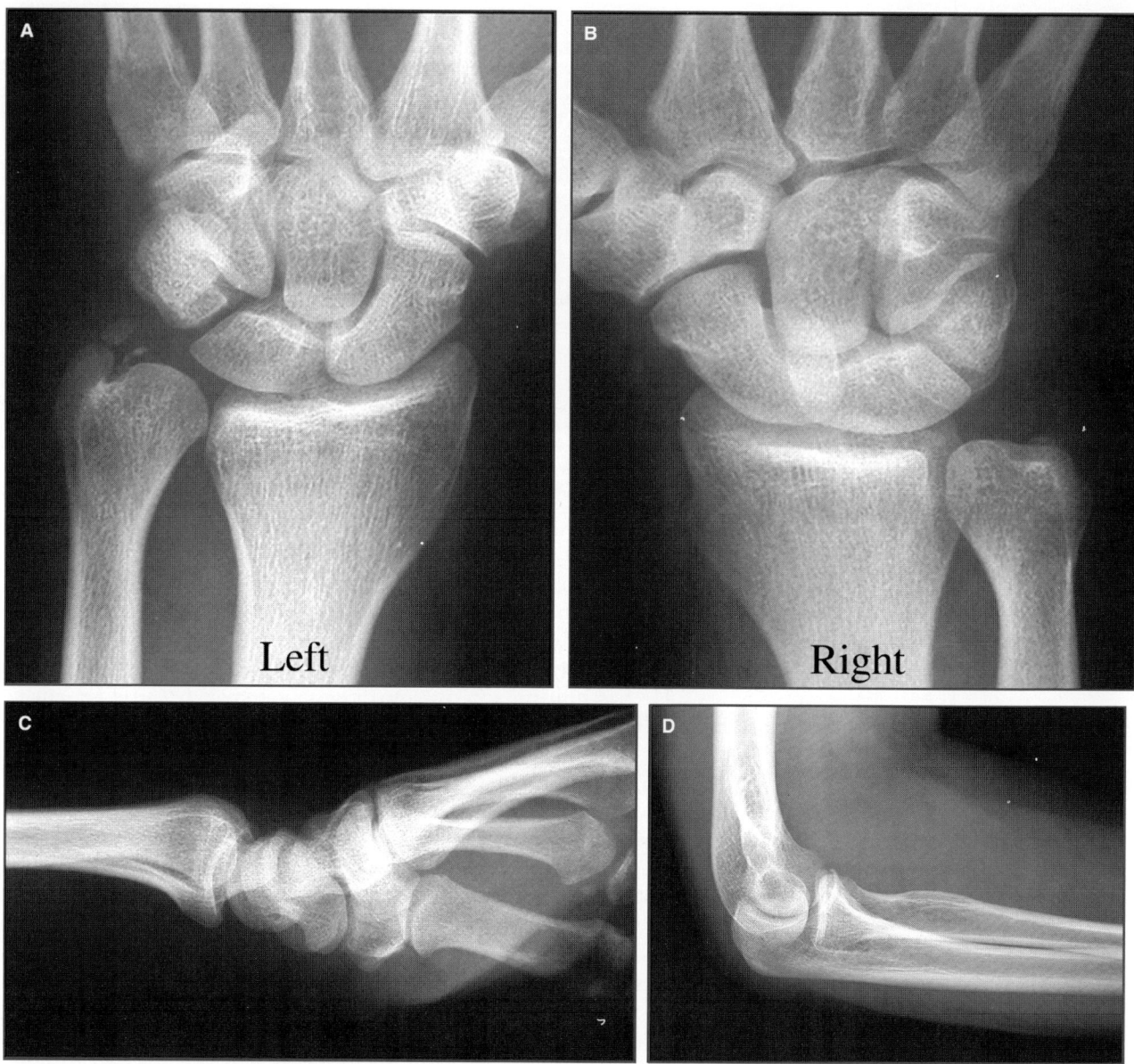

Figure 1 A and **B,** Comparison PA radiographs reveal 5 mm of positive ulnar variance in the affected wrist (left) and neutral variance in the opposite unaffected wrist (right). **C,** The lateral radiograph reveals a well-aligned DRUJ. **D,** A lateral view of the elbow was obtained to rule out associated radial head pathology or Essex-Lopresti injury.

have led to improved techniques and implants for reduction and fixation of the distal radius, ulnar-sided injuries of the wrist joint after fracture remain less well understood. Because of the inability to clearly define which fractures are predisposed to long-term instability or pain in this area, surgical indications are unclear. As a result, a conservative approach to treatment, specifically application of a long arm cast in the position of stability, closed reduction and percutaneous pinning of the ulna to the radius just proximal to the joint, and even routine open reduction and internal fixation of ulnar styloid fractures, has been recommended. Although most patients experience few to no long-term problems at the DRUJ after a wrist fracture, ulnar-sided pain and instability can result in significant disability for patients with these symptoms. Ulnar-sided symptoms have been implicated as the principal factor associated with poor outcomes after treatment of a wrist fracture.[1]

Part of the problem is that the anatomy of the DRUJ is very complex, and there are multiple structures responsible for stability and normal function. The articulation between the ulnar head and the sigmoid notch has some intrinsic stability, but it is a fairly loose joint with a combined rotation and gliding translation of the radius about the ulna. The axis of this motion is located at the base of the ulnar styloid in the foveal region of the distal ulna. Although most of the distal radioulnar ligaments and the triangular disk originate from this foveal location, these structures also may partially originate off of the base of the ulnar styloid. The subsheath of the extensor carpi ulnaris (ECU) and the volar ulnocarpal ligaments also are believed to add important stabilizing forces, and both have relationships with the styloid rather than the fovea.

The exact role that an ulnar styloid fracture plays in the genesis of ulnar-sided symptoms after a wrist fracture, therefore, depends on the exact location of the fracture. Fractures at the tip of the ulnar styloid are less likely to result in incompetence of the major ligamentous origins, whereas fractures closer to the foveal region are more likely to result in significant disruptions of these stabilizing structures. Perhaps the biggest problem in this analysis is that all of these ulnar-sided ligamentous structures can be rendered incompetent by a displaced distal radius fracture, even when the ulnar styloid is found to be intact radiographically. As in most clinical scenarios, physical examination at the DRUJ must be correlated with radiographic findings.

The stabilizing role of these ligamentous structures constitutes only one function of the triangular fibrocartilage complex (TFCC), however, because the TFCC also serves a dual role as a load-bearing structure, transferring 20% or more of the load from the carpal bones to the distal forearm.[2] Slight loss of length through the radius after a wrist fracture can markedly overload this balance of force transfer at the distal radius and ulna. Therefore, derangement at the ulnar side of the wrist after a fracture can be a result of isolated instability (eg, subluxating distal ulna), isolated load-bearing deficiency (eg, central triangular fibrocartilage [TFC] tear or ulnar abutment), or a combination of both. To complicate matters, other etiologies, such as symptomatic ulnar styloid nonunion, capsular and soft-tissue contracture, articular incongruity, and ECU tendon inflammation, have been proposed as contributing causes of ulnar-sided pain after a wrist fracture.

Instability

The diagnosis of instability after a distal radius fracture can only rarely be made on the basis of the initial radiographs. Diastasis of the radioulnar joint or dorsal migration of the radial epiphyseal fragment and the ulnar styloid from the ulnar head are sometimes seen on plain radiographs. Much of the time, however, radiographs are not definitive, and clinical stress testing after surgical stabilization of the radius fracture is required to better assess DRUJ instability. Although this ballottement test has been described clearly, it is a subjective assessment at best.[3] These findings must always be correlated with the findings on examination of the opposite wrist because natural laxity at the DRUJ is quite variable. This examination also should be performed with the forearm both maximally pronated and supinated. Instability after a wrist fracture is more typically identified when the forearm is pronated.

Clinical and Radiographic Assessment

Most patients present with instability symptoms after the distal radius fracture has healed. Patients with symptomatic instability of the DRUJ usually describe some combination of pain and abnormal motion on the ulnar side of the wrist. Crepitus or clicking with forearm rotation are typical findings, and the patient may even report that in certain positions the wrist is "out of joint" and needs to be manually reduced. Ballottement of the DRUJ should be performed. Careful palpation of the surrounding structures is essential to help define the precise location of any associated pain.

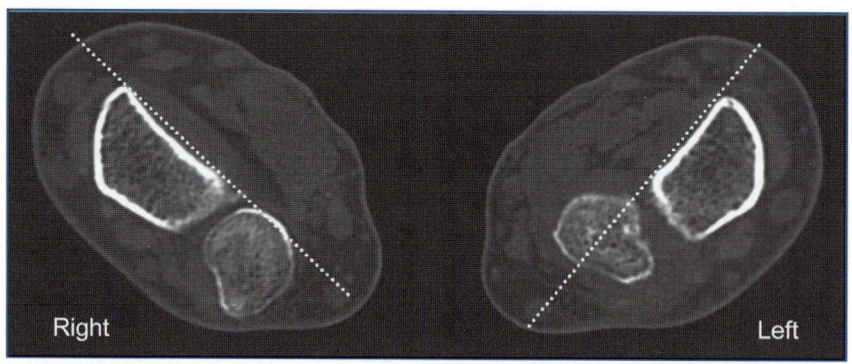

Figure 2 Comparison CT scans in supination. Note that the left wrist exhibits a volarly prominent ulnar head.

Pain in the ulnar snuffbox is typically associated with a TFC tear, whereas symptoms with manipulation of the carpal bones may indicate carpal instability. Pain at the tip of the styloid or along the ECU tendon is more indicative of tendon irritation or symptomatic nonunion at the site of the ulnar styloid than of true instability. Clinical examination is often quite limited in the acute setting, making assessment of the DRUJ problematic when treating wrist fractures in a cast. The DRUJ cannot be stressed until the fracture has healed or is rigidly fixed. Even in the subacute setting, when the fracture is healing and immobilization has been discontinued, the DRUJ is more difficult to assess because of the typical stiffness and decreased range of motion or pain that limits a full examination.

Although a true lateral radiograph can show subluxation or dislocation of the DRUJ, most patients with instability will have limited findings on radiographs. Comparative bilateral CT of the wrists is generally the most accurate means to identify static instability[4] (**Figure 2**). A number of systems have been designed to quantify the displacement identified on a CT scan, but all have somewhat poor reliability.[5] The affected wrist must be compared to the opposite, normal side to determine the extent of instability. It is often remarkable how little articular contact occurs between the sigmoid notch and ulnar head in full rotation in a normal wrist as a result of the translation of the radius on the ulna; therefore, false-positive results have been described.[5] CT also can provide important information about the condition of the articular surfaces of the sigmoid notch and ulnar head that is not evident on plain radiographs (**Figure 3**). In a patient with obvious unilateral symptomatic instability on clinical examination, CT is generally unnecessary.

DRUJ instability represents a spectrum of injury, but some authors have defined specific stages based on the severity of injury to the soft-tissue constraints.[3,6] Although it often is difficult to assign a patient to a specific category, it is worthwhile to understand the classification system. The typical patient with a distal radius fracture can, therefore, be considered to have no instability, instability, a reducible dislocation, or an irreducible (complex) dislocation (**Figure 4**). We prefer to consider instability as either mild-to-moderate or severe. A patient with mild-to-moderate instability is considered to have increased displacement in only one direction and/or in one position of testing, typically dorsal displacement of the ulna in the pronated position. Severe instability is marked displacement in both directions and in all forearm positions.

Treatment of the Acute Injury

After stabilization of the radius fracture, clinical findings must be compared with those of the opposite, normal wrist. Clearly, in a patient with no appreciable DRUJ instability, isolated treatment of the distal radius fracture is sufficient. For patients with mild instability, casting or splinting that immobilizes the forearm in a neutral position usually is acceptable because the laxity generally is the result of an incomplete disruption of the DRUJ-stabilizing structures. Casting or splinting allows for adequate healing of the soft-tissue envelope. Six weeks of immobilization followed by active and then passive motion generally adequately restores motion and stability to the DRUJ. Some consideration can be given to immobilization in

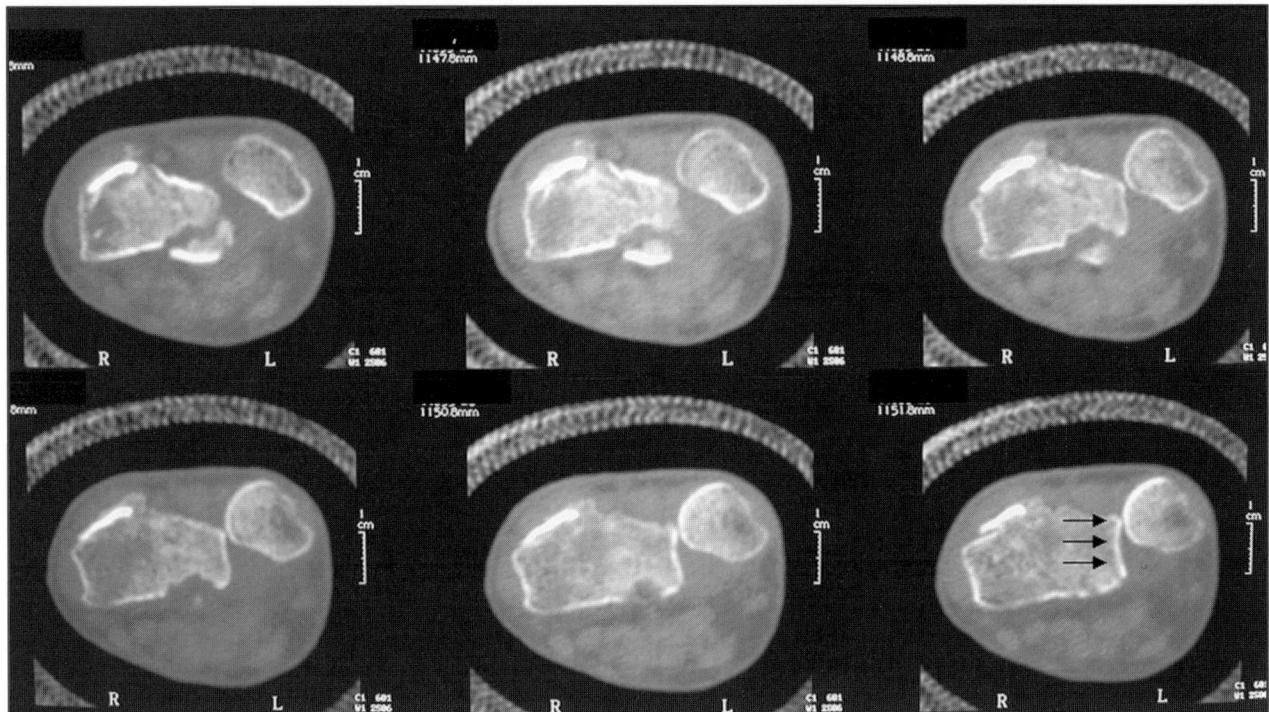

Figure 3 Postreduction CT scans of a 43-year-old woman who fractured her wrist in a fall while rollerblading. Note that there is some mild dorsal translation of the distal ulna on the lower three images and a displaced volar ulnar sigmoid notch fragment on the upper three images.

the position of maximal stability if the laxity on clinical examination is believed to be moderate, but still in only one testing position. A possible disadvantage to the latter approach is stiffness in this maximally rotated position that may require extensive physical therapy or even further surgery. Pinning of the forearm in neutral rotation after reduction of the ulnar head is a reliable procedure for moderate instability, especially for patients who are presumed to be noncompliant with braces or casts that limit forearm rotation.

In patients with more severe instability or a reducible dislocation, acute surgical repair of the torn TFCC should be considered (**Figure 5**). Fixation of a torn TFCC or ulnar styloid is not a simple procedure given the traumatic disruption of ulnar wrist anatomy, the limited exposure to the joint, and the often small size of the styloid fragment. However, repair of the TFCC at the time of distal radius fixation is a much more straightforward procedure than a late repair when scarring and ligament retraction signifi-

cantly complicate the procedure.[7] We believe that in the patient with gross instability of the DRUJ, simple pinning of the reduced DRUJ may be ill advised. Although closed reduction of the ulnar head into the sigmoid notch secured with Kirschner wires (K-wires) from the ulna into the radius generally appears acceptable on plain radiographs, the TFCC origin, the ulnar styloid, and the entire soft-tissue envelope may remain at a distance from their actual anatomic origins, even with the ulnar head located within the notch. In this situation, the ulnar styloid and TFCC are unlikely to heal properly, and the DRUJ is predisposed to late instability when the pins are removed and physical therapy initiated.

After repair of the styloid and/or TFCC for severe DRUJ instability, pinning of the forearm bones to augment stability is based on the degree of soft-tissue disruption. Because insertion of a 1.6-mm pin from the ulna across to the radius just proximal to the DRUJ has associated complications, pinning should

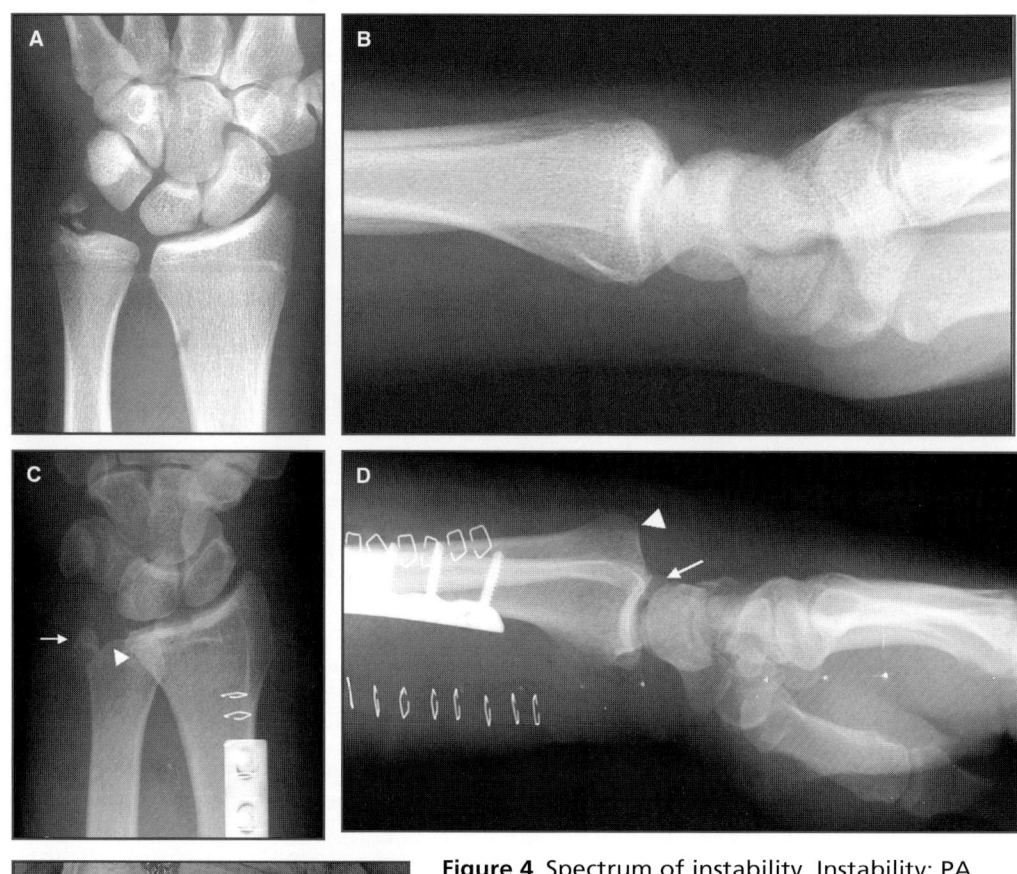

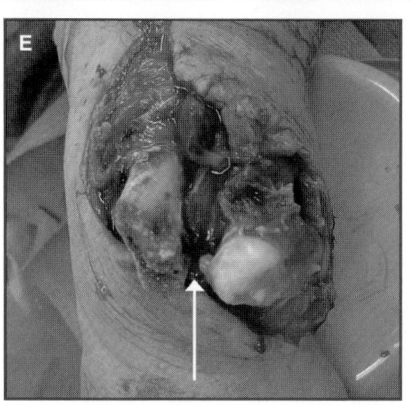

Figure 4 Spectrum of instability. Instability: PA **(A)** and lateral **(B)** radiographs showing styloid nonunion. Both views appear normal, but the patient reports symptoms of instability. Reducible dislocation: PA **(C)** and lateral **(D)** radiographs of a dorsally dislocated distal ulna after a Galeazzi fracture and nondisplaced marginal volar lip fracture. The arrowhead identifies the normal anatomic position of the styloid base; the arrow illustrates the degree of styloid displacement. Irreducible dislocation: Intraoperative photograph **(E)** demonstrating gross deformity and soft-tissue interposition. The arrow identifies the entire wrist extensor tendon mass entrapped in the DRUJ.

be avoided if possible (**Figure 6**). In general, pinning should be used only to augment styloid or TFCC repair. Positioning the pins across all four cortices simplifies removal if a pin breaks. We often place two pins in a large adult to reduce the likelihood of pin breakage. If the styloid is securely fixed after an avulsion of the styloid base, and disruption of the adjacent capsule tissue is securely reapproximated, then pinning the radius to the ulna is generally omitted, and the forearm is splinted in a neutral position (**Figure 5,** C and D).

For patients with a distal radius fracture and an irreducible dislocation of the DRUJ, open reduction and fixation of the TFCC and/or ulnar styloid is man-

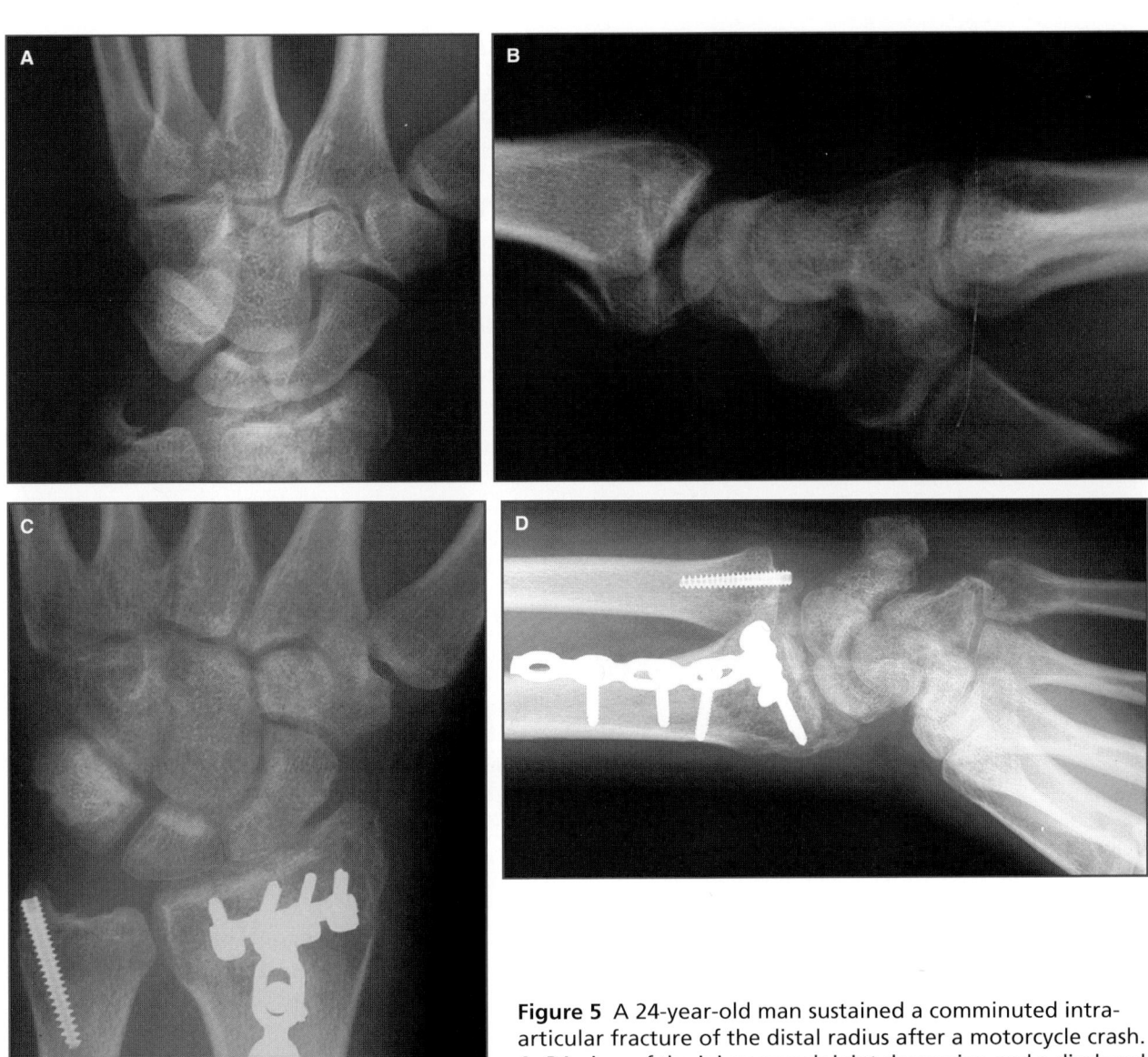

Figure 5 A 24-year-old man sustained a comminuted intra-articular fracture of the distal radius after a motorcycle crash. **A,** PA view of the injury reveals joint depression and a displaced ulnar styloid fracture that encompasses the entire base of the styloid and the fovea. **B,** The lateral view reveals volar carpal subluxation, joint impaction, and a reduced DRUJ. After fixation of the radius, the DRUJ was found to be quite unstable, with complete disruption of the surrounding DRUJ capsule. PA **(C)** and lateral **(D)** radiographs of the healed radius and ulnar styloid after open reduction and internal fixation with a headless screw. Clinical stability was excellent.

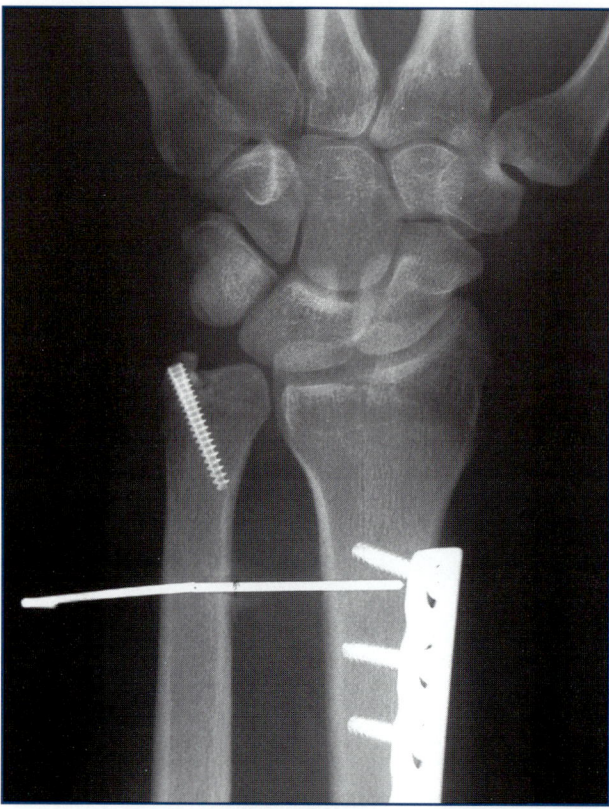

Figure 6 PA radiograph reveals pin failure with retraction into the ulnar shaft 5 weeks after ulnar styloid repair and DRUJ pinning. The patient required an additional operation for pin removal.

datory (**Figure 7**). It is not uncommon for these severe dislocations to be associated with an open injury of the DRUJ and/or the distal radius fracture; therefore, irrigation and débridement must occur before the fracture and dislocation are addressed. Entrapment of the ulnar head buttonholed within adjacent musculotendinous or capsular structures, interposition of flexor or extensor tendons within the joint, and simple entrapment of the torn and rotated TFCC between the ulnar head and sigmoid notch have been described as causes of the irreducible dislocation. Once the ulnar head has been reduced into the notch, repair of the ulnar styloid or TFCC complex can proceed and is generally augmented with pins across the forearm bones for 6 to 8 weeks to allow sufficient healing before beginning physical therapy.

Ulnar Styloid Repair

Our preferred approach for acute fixation involves a longitudinal incision along the subcutaneous border of the distal ulna. This incision generally is located at a safe distance from either a dorsal or volar incision for the distal radius fracture, resulting in an adequate skin bridge. Care must be taken to identify and protect the dorsal sensory branch of the ulnar nerve. Exposure of the styloid fragment is generally adequate with this approach and allows for a complete assessment of the extent of disruption of the DRUJ capsule and ECU subsheath, as well as visualization of the head of the distal ulna. It is imperative to determine that the bulk of the TFCC is attached to the styloid while minimizing dissection around the styloid fragment to prevent loss of continuity of these essential ligaments. The TFCC almost always remains attached to a larger ulnar styloid fragment; therefore, realignment of the complex can be anticipated with reduction of the styloid fragment.

After débridement and irrigation of the hematoma and any interposed periosteum from the fracture surface on the distal ulna, a piercing clip is placed around the styloid fragment and used to reduce the styloid to the ulna; internal fixation of the styloid is then performed. If a tension-band technique is selected, two 0.035-in K-wires are usually the right size to fit into the fragment and are directed into the metaphysis of the distal ulna. Next, 24-gauge wire is wrapped around the exposed K-wire and through a bone tunnel created in the proximal fragment. The wire is tensioned, the K-wires are backed out slightly, bent, and cut, then gently impacted until flush with the deep soft tissues (**Figure 8, _A_**).

When a larger styloid fragment is identified, we prefer fixation of the fragment with a cannulated headless screw. The surgical approach is the same, but the styloid fragment is pinned with a small guide wire into the distal ulnar metaphysis. A cannulated drill prepares the bone tunnel, then an 18- to 24-mm screw is advanced across the fracture (**Figure 8, _B_**). Compression is excellent, although care must be taken to control for fragment rotation during final screw insertion. This construct is extremely stable and, because the screw head is buried, does not require screw removal. Fragmentation of the styloid during insertion must be prevented; therefore, we avoid this technique for small styloid fragments or smaller patients.

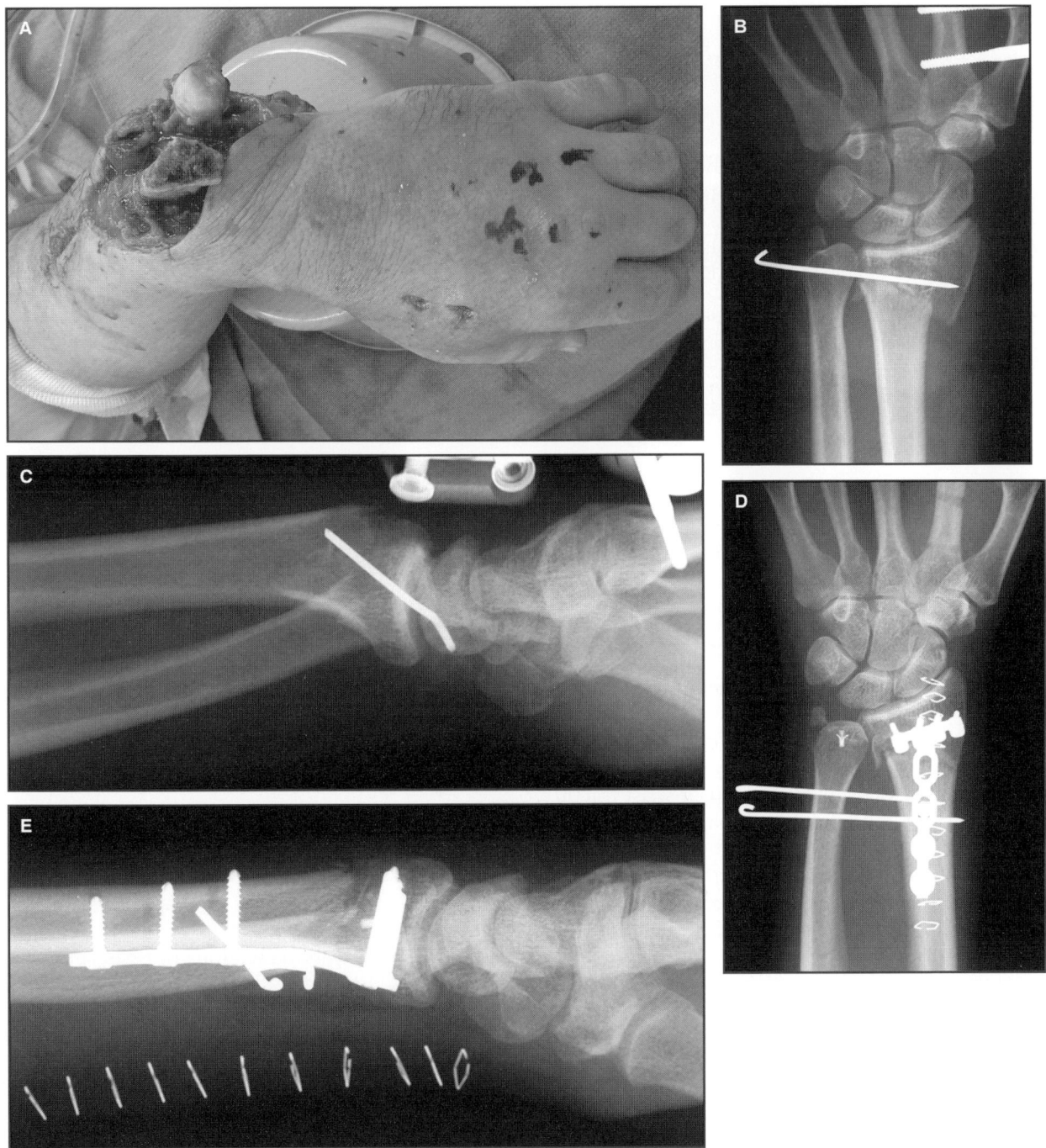

Figure 7 A, Intraoperative photograph of an open wrist fracture/DRUJ dislocation in a 42-year-old man involved in a motorcycle crash. The wound was thoroughly irrigated, a temporary external fixator was applied, and a single K-wire was placed to stabilize the DRUJ after open reduction. **B,** PA radiograph after initial treatment reveals persistent displacement of both radial and ulnar styloid fragments. **C,** The lateral view reveals marked rotatory malposition of the distal radius but reduction of the DRUJ. PA **(D)** and lateral **(E)** views after definitive fixation with a locked volar plate and suture anchor fixation of the TFCC to the ulnar fovea. The DRUJ was pinned in a slightly supinated position.

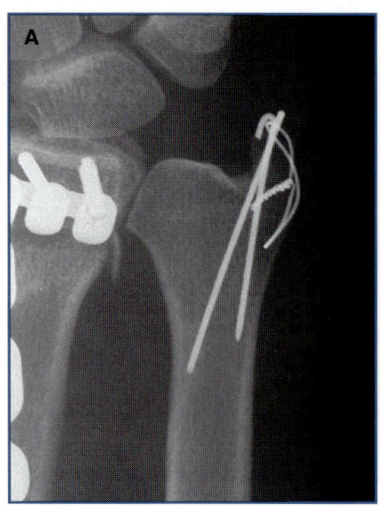
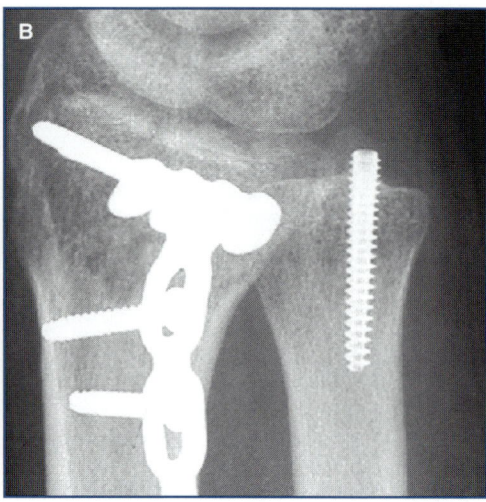

Figure 8 Postoperative radiographs of tension-band technique **(A)** and headless compression screw technique **(B)** for treatment of displaced unstable ulnar styloid fractures after distal radius fixation.

Treatment of Late Injury

For patients with a healed, well-aligned distal radius fracture and clinical instability at the DRUJ, a careful physical examination and wrist radiographs are required to rule out associated injuries to nearby structures. Wrist arthrography and/or CT or high-resolution MRI also can help identify associated lesions. Repair of the ulnar styloid nonunion or excision of a small styloid fragment and repair of the TFCC back to the ulnar fovea generally is appropriate in symptomatic patients within a year of wrist fracture. For patients who present more than 1 year after the fracture, the ability to advance these attenuated or partially healed structures back to their true origin becomes uncertain. It is impossible to say at what point repair of the TFCC should be converted to formal reconstruction. Some authors report good results from repair of the TFCC or ulnar styloid 5 years or more after injury,[8] whereas others report converting to a formal reconstruction of the TFCC as little as 4 months after the original injury.[9] The safest approach for this type of patient is to attempt repair if possible; however, knowledge of the technique of, and informed consent for, ligamentous reconstruction is advised.

In a patient with a distal radius malunion, the looseness associated with DRUJ instability on clinical examination often improves or resolves with correction of distal radius anatomy by osteotomy. If normal ulnar variance has not been restored (based on a comparison view of the opposite wrist), ulnar shortening also should be considered. In a patient with normal ulnar variance and a well-aligned distal radius, the ulnar styloid nonunion or the TFCC can be repaired to its origin. If tissue quality does not allow for this repair, ligament reconstruction at the DRUJ is appropriate. The longer the patient has had instability symptoms, the more likely reconstruction will be required.

DRUJ Ligament Reconstruction

A variety of nonanatomic DRUJ reconstruction procedures have been replaced by anatomic reconstructions of the DRUJ described recently by a number of authors.[9,10] The basic tenet of anatomic reconstruction involves restoration of the palmar and dorsal radioulnar ligaments via tendon graft passed through drill holes in the distal radius and ulna. We perform a complete arthroscopic examination of the wrist intraoperatively to address other intra-articular pathology and to help identify articular derangement that could predispose a patient to a worse outcome.

A dorsal longitudinal incision is centered over the DRUJ. The fifth compartment is opened, and the ulnar aspect of the fourth compartment is elevated subperiosteally off of the radius for clear identification. The DRUJ capsule is released from the dorsal aspect of the sigmoid notch, and the capsular incision is extended across the dorsal ulnocarpal capsule, creating an L-shaped capsular flap that can be retracted ulnarly. This exposes the DRUJ and TFC, although elevation of the base of the sixth compartment off of the distal ulna is minimized. A second incision, made on the volar side of the wrist centered over the flexor carpi ulnaris (FCU), is used for volar exposure. The sigmoid notch and volar aspect of the radius can be approached by ulnar retraction of the FCU and ulnar neurovascular bundle. The ulnar shaft is exposed by radial retraction of these same structures.

A cannulated drill system is used to recreate the anatomic origins of the dorsal and palmar distal radioulnar ligaments while avoiding penetration of the sigmoid notch and the lunate facet of the distal radius. A tunnel between 4.0 and 4.5 mm in diameter generally is required for passage of the graft, and caution must be exercised to avoid fracture of the bone bridge. We use a 28-gauge wire folded over once to pass the graft through the bone tunnels. Once the graft has been passed through the bone tunnel in the radius, both limbs of the graft are passed through a bone tunnel in the ulna connecting the fovea to the ulnar shaft. To create this tunnel, the cannulated drill guidewire is passed retrograde from the foveal insertion point out the medial border of the ulna. The cannulated drill bit is then passed over the guidewire, drilling anterograde from the medial border of the ulna toward the fovea to avoid difficulty with the passage of the rigid drill bit across the dorsum of the wrist. Because both limbs of the graft are passed through this tunnel, it may need to be widened another millimeter or two by sequential drilling with larger drill bits.

The two limbs of the graft are then passed back across the dorsal and volar surfaces of the distal ulna, woven through the remaining DRUJ capsule, and secured to the limbs of the graft near the sigmoid notch margin. The graft is tensioned with the forearm in neutral rotation and the radius and ulna compressed together manually. Pinning of the DRUJ is optional, and we prefer to avoid it in a compliant patient. A rigid sugar-tong splint is applied for 10 days and converted to a Muenster cast for a total of 6 weeks immobilization. A removable splint replaces the cast, and physical therapy is initiated. Motion is limited to active and active-assist motion for the first 2 weeks after cast removal, and gripping or lifting activities are prohibited for at least 3 months after surgery. Progressive passive stretching and/or splinting can be in-

TABLE 1 Sources of Ulnar-sided Pain

TFCC tears
DRUJ instability
Lunotriquetral interosseous ligament tears/instability
Ulnar abutment/impaction
Proximal hamate arthrosis
Contracture DRUJ capsule
Chondromalacia/osteoarthritis at DRUJ or lunate fossa
ECU tendinitis/subluxation
Cutaneous neuroma
Ulnar styloid nonunion
Pisotriquetral osteoarthritis
Reflex sympathetic dystrophy

troduced at 8 weeks to address any deficiencies in motion.

Ulnar-sided Wrist Pain

Ulnar-sided wrist pain is common after healing of a distal radius fracture. The list of possible causes is extensive (**Table 1**), and in some patients complete resolution of symptoms may not be possible. A careful history to elicit the location of the pain and any exacerbating motions or activities is critical to narrow the differential diagnosis. A careful physical examination that localizes maximal pain and documents any DRUJ or carpal instability further narrows the differential diagnosis. The use of radiography, arthrography, and/or CT and MRI clearly depends on the presumed source of the pathology. Patients may have more than one source of pathology after a distal radius fracture.

Treatment of ulnar-sided wrist pain after distal radius fracture clearly depends on the underlying etiology. TFCC tears are common after wrist fractures, with an incidence of 50% or more, and seem to be correlated with the initial degree of displacement and angulation of the bone fragments at the time of injury.[11-13] Although arthrography or MRI can be used to identify these tears, wrist arthroscopy remains the gold standard for diagnosis. Palmer[14] classified these tears based on the acuity and location of the tear (**Table 2**), and treatment clearly depends on its location.

A number of studies have explored the utility of

TABLE 2 Palmer Classification of TFCC Tears

Type I Acute tears

    IA Central linear tear

    IB Ulnar peripheral tear

    IC Volar ulnar carpal ligament tear

    ID Radial-sided tears/avulsions

Type II Chronic tears/ulnar impaction

    IIA Central linear tear

    IIB Ulnar peripheral tear

    IIC Volar ulnar carpal ligament tear

    IID Radial-sided tears/avulsion

wrist arthroscopy in identifying and classifying TFCC tears at the time of wrist fracture, but the benefit of arthroscopic treatment of these soft-tissue injuries at the time of fracture is unknown.[12,13] In general, most wrist fractures are treated primarily for the bony injury without arthroscopy; the soft-tissue injury is addressed surgically only if instability is identified radiographically or clinically at the time of fracture stabilization. By convention, patients with a TFCC tear are treated only after they report persistent pain after fracture healing and a period of physical therapy; treatment generally is arthroscopic. It remains to be seen whether arthroscopic treatment of these TFCC injuries at the time the wrist fracture is treated actually reduces the incidence of symptoms after the fracture has healed.

Central linear TFCC tears, type IA, are not common after wrist fracture but when present they are easily visualized with arthroscopy. Many of the central tears found during arthroscopy are probably the result of degenerative wear and may even predate the fracture. Degenerative central tears in the setting of a healed wrist fracture where the radius has settled 1 mm or more represent the common Palmer type IIC chronic tear. Both type IA and type IIC tears usually are adequately treated by arthroscopic débridement. A combination of shavers, punches, and thermal ablators can be used to adequately resect loose flaps of the central tear back to stable dorsal and volar margins. Some consideration should be given to wafer resection or formal ulnar shortening if symptoms develop a year or more after fracture healing or if the associated changes of ulnar impaction are present. These signs include (1) radiographic cystic changes in

the carpal bones or ulnar head, (2) chondromalacia of the carpal bones, or (3) a lunotriquetral interosseus ligament tear.

The true incidence of type IB peripheral tears after wrist fracture is unclear and seems to depend on the definition. Ulnar styloid fractures are present in 50% to 70% of wrist fractures,[1,13] and if the foveal ligamentous attachments are displaced with the styloid, this fracture is a variant of a type IB tear. However, there also is a subset of patients without a styloid fracture and with an arthroscopically diagnosed peripheral tear.[11] These findings illustrate the importance of determining whether an ulnar styloid fragment is associated with DRUJ instability at the time of fracture fixation but also emphasize that fixation of an ulnar styloid fragment is less important than ensuring that the peripheral attachments of the TFCC are firmly secured to their foveal insertion.

In patients with ulnar-sided wrist pain who present after fracture healing and a period of physical therapy, and in whom either no or mild instability is detected, arthroscopic-assisted or open repair of the ulnar rim of the TFCC is advised.[8,15] Arthroscopic débridement of the peripheral capsule preceding arthroscopic suture insertion into the dorsal and volar rim allows for accurate placement of the sutures. However, it is advisable to clearly identify the ulnar capsule through a small open incision before tying the knots of these sutures to ensure that neurovascular and tendinous structures are not incorporated into the repair. If the patient has a type IB tear with an ulnar styloid nonunion, formal open excision of the bone fragment with direct repair of the TFCC to the surrounding capsule and/or bone via tunnels or suture anchors is our standard approach.

Type IC tears are treated at the time of wrist fracture by immobilizing the fracture. The volar ulnar carpal ligaments are torn in only 5% of fractures and are likely to heal acceptably in most patients because of the close apposition of the torn ends with wrist immobilization.[13] Long-term difficulties from poor healing of these ligaments remain an unsolved and uncommon problem, and the literature contains no clear treatment guidelines.

By comparison, type ID tears are quite common after distal radius fractures.[12,13] These tears often occur with bony avulsion of the ligamentous origin at the sigmoid notch (**Figure 3**). For tears identified at the time of fracture, nonsurgical treatment after stabilization of the radius fracture is adequate in most patients. The only clear exception is a patient with a large displaced bone fragment at the corner of the lunate facet that can be surgically reduced and stabilized either via sutures or screws.

When patients present with pain after the wrist fracture has healed, and a type ID radial margin tear is diagnosed, arthroscopic débridement will reliably improve symptoms. However, this approach may result in long-term loss of the load-bearing properties of the TFCC. Repair of the TFCC back to its radial origin seems more promising; however, retraction of the torn TFCC edge and the poor vascularity of the radial margin of the disk complicate this surgery. In our experience, arthroscopic and open repairs have had acceptable results but are performed only in a young patient within 1 or 2 years of the initial injury.[15]

Ulnar-sided wrist pain after healing of a distal radius fracture can sometimes be a misleading symptom. When a patient describes "pain" and/or "aching" on the ulnar side of the wrist, it is important to determine whether the patient's problem actually is loss of motion at the DRUJ and the pain associated with trying to improve it. Kleinman and Graham[16] investigated this condition and showed that release of the DRUJ capsule in the setting of a well-aligned distal radius can improve motion and decrease pain.

Pain on the ulnar side of the wrist after fracture healing can also result from degenerative changes at the DRUJ. Whether caused by articular incongruity or by impaction of the cartilage surfaces at the time of injury and resultant chondrocyte death, this condition is significantly more problematic to resolve. If nonsurgical modalities, such as nonsteroidal anti-inflammatory drugs or splinting, no longer provide significant relief, surgical treatment should be undertaken cautiously. The Darrach procedure was originally described for DRUJ degeneration and/or instability after wrist fracture,[17] and although it has proved reliable in a number of patient populations, some results have not been as favorable.[18] Despite attempts to create tendon or fascial slings to support the remaining ulnar stump, instability and persistent ulnar-sided pain have led some to abandon this procedure in a postfracture population. Its one true indication may remain in the elderly or extremely low-demand patient for whom pain relief, rather than gripping and lifting function, is the principal goal.

The Bowers' hemiresection interposition procedure,[19] the Watson's matched resection,[20] and the Sauvé-Kapandji procedure[21] were introduced in response to the inconsistent results of the Darrach resection in a high-demand patient. Although each procedure has been shown to be somewhat helpful for treating the symptoms of a degenerative DRUJ, all can result in postoperative instability and/or impingement, and all three remain an incomplete solution. Because of the frequency of incomplete relief or failure, we try to avoid these procedures. If the patient's primary problem and source of pain is DRUJ instability, then these resection and pseudarthrosis procedures are highly contraindicated; a ligament reconstruction and/or ulnar shortening is the procedure of choice. Furthermore, for most patients presenting with a typically shortened and dorsally tilted distal radius malunion and ulnar-sided wrist pain, corrective osteotomy of the radius is a much more sensible procedure than resection of all or a portion of the prominent distal ulna.

MANAGEMENT AND OUTCOME SUMMARY

Our case example presents the history and physical findings of a patient with severe instability of the DRUJ who presented almost 8 years after the fracture. Stress examination of the DRUJ revealed both dorsal and palmar instability of the distal ulna in all testing positions, which was significantly different from the opposite normal wrist. Although radiographs revealed good alignment of the distal radial articular surface, comparison to the opposite wrist revealed a 5-mm increase in ulnar variance (**Figure 1**). This clinical outcome from such a minimally displaced fracture is somewhat atypical and, therefore, prevention of this outcome would have been difficult. However, this case certainly underscores the importance of vigilance for ulnar-sided pathology after wrist fractures and careful examination of patients who present with persistent ulnar-sided symptoms after a period of fracture healing and physical therapy.

This patient's problems were twofold. First, the instability of the DRUJ was symptomatic and needed to be addressed. Second, because of the length of time from the original fracture to present treatment, changes consistent with ulnar impaction within the

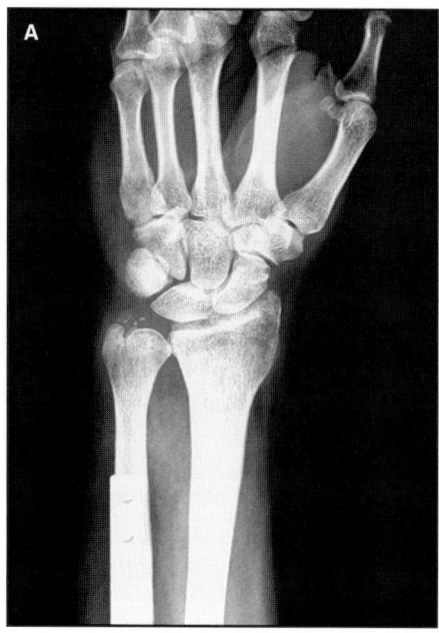

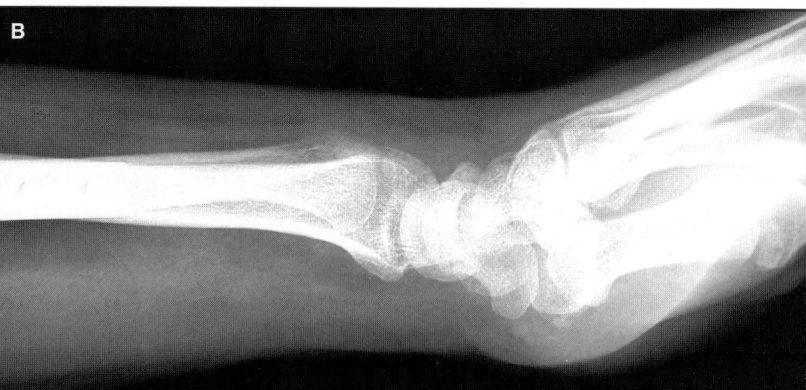

Figure 9 Postoperative radiographs of the patient shown in **Figure 1**. PA **(A)** and lateral **(B)** radiographs after a 5-mm ulnar shortening procedure reveal restoration of neutral ulnar variance and a reduced DRUJ.

ulnar aspect of the wrist were likely contributing to the patient's clinical symptoms. Any surgical treatment must, therefore, address these problems concomitantly. Realignment of the DRUJ with either a shortening osteotomy of the ulna or lengthening of the radius would accomplish two objectives. Realigning the ulnar head within the sigmoid notch and retensioning the ulnar-sided soft-tissue restraints should lead to improvements in DRUJ stability and reduction in ulnar impaction symptoms. Ulnar shortening seems simpler in this situation; it is contraindicated only in the presence of more obvious radial deformity. Incomplete restoration of stability is possible even after realignment, however. Additional procedures for stabilization of the DRUJ may be required, and the patient should be counseled about this possibility.

After discussion of the expected benefits and possible risks from ulnar shortening and fixation, and possible DRUJ repair or reconstruction, the patient elected to undergo surgery. An ulnar-sided subcutaneous approach to the distal third of the ulna was used. The interval between the FCU and ECU muscles was used to expose the volar ulnar surface. A seven-hole plate was positioned over the distal third of the ulna and secured with the two distal screws. The site of the oblique osteotomy was marked and the plate removed. Five millimeters of bone was then excised us-

ing parallel cuts of an oscillating saw under constant saline irrigation. The plate was reapplied distally, and the osteotomy was compressed and remaining screws placed. The middle hole of the plate was used for lag screw placement. Radiographs revealed restoration of neutral ulnar variance (**Figure 9**).

After the shortening was completed, manual stress testing of the DRUJ revealed marked improvement. Clinically, the laxity was still increased compared with the opposite wrist, but pathologic subluxation of the distal ulna was no longer seen in either the dorsal or palmar direction. Therefore, TFCC repair or reconstruction was not performed. The patient was placed in a sugar-tong splint intraoperatively and converted to a Muenster cast at the first postoperative visit for a total of 6 weeks immobilization. Physical therapy was initiated at the time of cast removal, and the patient returned to the clinic after 3 months with 80% resolution of his initial clinical complaints. The patient was asked to consider wrist arthroscopy and DRUJ repair or reconstruction if residual symptoms persisted or worsened. Six months later, the patient has not returned.

As evident from this case, the assessment of the DRUJ after a wrist fracture can be quite challenging. Frequently, both the physical examination and plain radiographs are equivocal, or worse yet, more than one problem may exist. Treatment recommendations for the acute fracture with marked instability are quite clear and focus on restoration of ligamentous continuity. Reconstruction for the subacute or chronic condition must be undertaken cautiously, and a step-wise approach (as performed in this case) is often valuable. Much like the situation in this case, it is important to consider both the ligamentous and load-bearing properties of the structures forming the DRUJ when making treatment decisions. Clearly identifying the symptoms as instability and/or pain also allows clear differentiation of the likely causes and helps guide correct treatment. Reconstruction of normal anatomy is generally preferred in most situations, with bony procedures generally performed before ligament repairs or reconstructions. Salvage-type distal ulnar ablation procedures should be avoided as much as possible and reserved for patients with joint degeneration in the face of near-normal DRUJ anatomy and stability.

REFERENCES

1. Knirk JL, Jupiter JB: Intra-articular fractures of the distal end of the radius in young adults. *J Bone Joint Surg Am* 1986;68:647-659.

2. Palmer AK, Werner FW: Biomechanics of the distal radioulnar joint. *Clin Orthop* 1984;187:26-35.

3. Cheng SL, Axelrod TS: Management of complex dislocations of the distal radioulnar joint. *Clin Orthop* 1997;341:183-191.

4. Mino DE, Palmer AK, Levinsohn EM: Radiography and computerized tomography in the diagnosis of incongruity of the distal radioulnar joint. *J Bone Joint Surg Am* 1985;67:247-252.

5. Pan C, Lin Y, Lee T, Chou C: Displacement of the distal radioulnar joint of the clinically symptom free patients. *Clin Orthop* 2003;415:148-156.

6. Bruckner JD, Lichtman DM, Alexander AH: Complex dislocations of the distal radioulnar joint: Recognition and management. *Clin Orthop* 1992;275:90-103.

7. Nicolaidis SC, Hildreth DH, Lichtman DM: Acute injuries of the distal radioulnar joint. *Hand Clinics* 2000;16:449-459.

8. Hauck RM, Skahen J III, Palmer AK: Classification and treatment of ulnar styloid nonunion. *J Hand Surg [Am]* 1996;21:418-422.

9. Adams BD, Berger RA: An anatomic reconstruction of the distal radioulnar ligaments for posttraumatic distal radioulnar joint instability. *J Hand Surg [Am]* 2002;27:243-251.

10. Henry, MH, Smith DW, Masson MV: Reconstruction of distal radioulnar joint instability. *J Am Soc Surg Hand* 2004;4:35-41.

11. Geissler WB, Freeland AE, Savoie FH, McIntyre LW, Whipple TL: Intracarpal soft-tissue lesions associated with an intra-articular fracture of the distal end of the radius. *J Bone Joint Surg Am* 1996;78:357-365.

12. Mehta JA, Bain GI, Heptinstall RJ: Anatomical reduction of intra-articular fractures of the distal radius: An arthroscopically assisted approach. *J Bone Joint Surg Br* 2000;82:79-86.

13. Richards RS, Bennett JD, Roth JH, Milne K Jr: Arthroscopic diagnosis of intra-articular soft tissue injuries associated with distal radial fractures. *J Hand Surg [Am]* 1997;22:772-776.

14. Palmer AK: Triangular fibrocartilage complex lesions: A classification. *J Hand Surg [Am]* 1989;14:594-605.

15. Trumble TE, Gilbert M, Vedder N: Isolated tears of the triangular fibrocartilage: Management by early arthroscopic repair. *J Hand Surg [Am]* 1997;22:57-65.

16. Kleinman WB, Graham TJ: The distal radioulnar joint capsule: Clinical anatomy and role in post-traumatic limitation of forearm rotation. *J Hand Surg [Am]* 1998;23:588-599.

17. Darrach W: Fracture of the lower extremity of the radius: Diagnosis and treatment. *JAMA* 1927;89:1683-1685.

18. af Ekenstam F, Engkvist O, Wadin K: Results from resection of the distal end of the ulna after fractures of the lower end of the radius. *Scand J Plast Reconstr Surg* 1982;16:177-181.

19. Bowers WH: Distal radioulnar joint arthroplasty: The hemiresection-interposition technique. *J Hand Surg [Am]* 1985;10:169-178.

20. Watson HK, Ryu JY, Burgess RC: Matched distal ulnar resection. *J Hand Surg [Am]* 1986;11:812-817.

21. Sauvé L, Kapandji M: Une Nouvelle technique de traitement chirurgical des luxation récidivantes isolées de l'extrémité inferievre de cubitus. *J Chir* 1936;47:589-594.

STIFFNESS AND JOINT CONTRACTURE

F. Thomas D. Kaplan, MD

RADIOCARPAL STIFFNESS AND CONTRACTURE
Case Presentation

A 72-year-old retired executive who sustained a comminuted, extra-articular distal radius fracture and an ulnar neck fracture in a motor vehicle accident underwent closed reduction in the emergency department on the day of injury. Significant residual deformity (**Figure 1**) and the onset of paresthesias in the median nerve distribution noted on the postreduction examination indicated the need for surgical repair. Fracture fixation was performed that evening through a volar approach for the distal radius fracture and an ulnar approach for the ulnar neck fracture (**Figure 2**).

Ten days postoperatively, the patient had normal sensation in all digits without residual paresthesias. His initial wrist motion was 45° of extension, 20° of flexion, 50° of pronation, and 30° of supination. He also had full range of motion (ROM) in the fingers. Physical therapy was initiated with active, active-assist, and passive ROM exercises, and the patient was given a volar splint to be worn between exercise sessions. At his 6-week follow-up appointment, he had made modest improvements, with wrist extension of 55°, flexion of 35°, pronation of 60°, and supination of 35°.

Discussion
Clinical Assessment

Loss of motion following distal radius fracture is extremely common. Often, the patient has adequate function with the amount of remaining motion, and no further treatment is sought. However, in patients with significantly restricted motion or in higher-demand patients with less tolerance to stiffness, the residual disability from decreased ROM requires treatment. The amount of motion loss depends on multiple factors, including the characteristics of the fracture, associated injury, patient factors, and the type of treatment selected. Fortunately, patients often function well despite residual wrist stiffness.

Residual deformity of the joint is perhaps the most significant factor in predicting the recovery of motion. Articular incongruity results in progressive arthrosis and loss of motion, whereas increasing degrees of malunion limit the potential recovery of motion.[1,2] Dorsal angulation of the articular surface of the radius leads to a compensatory carpal flexion deformity and corresponding

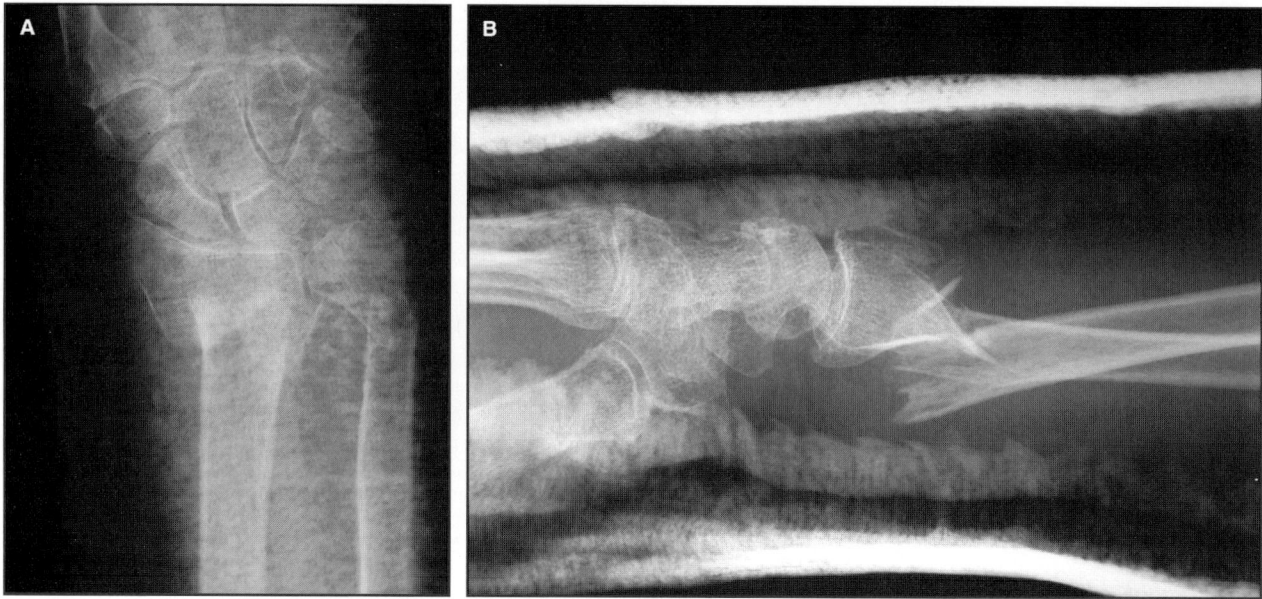

Figure 1 PA **(A)** and lateral **(B)** radiographs after reduction.

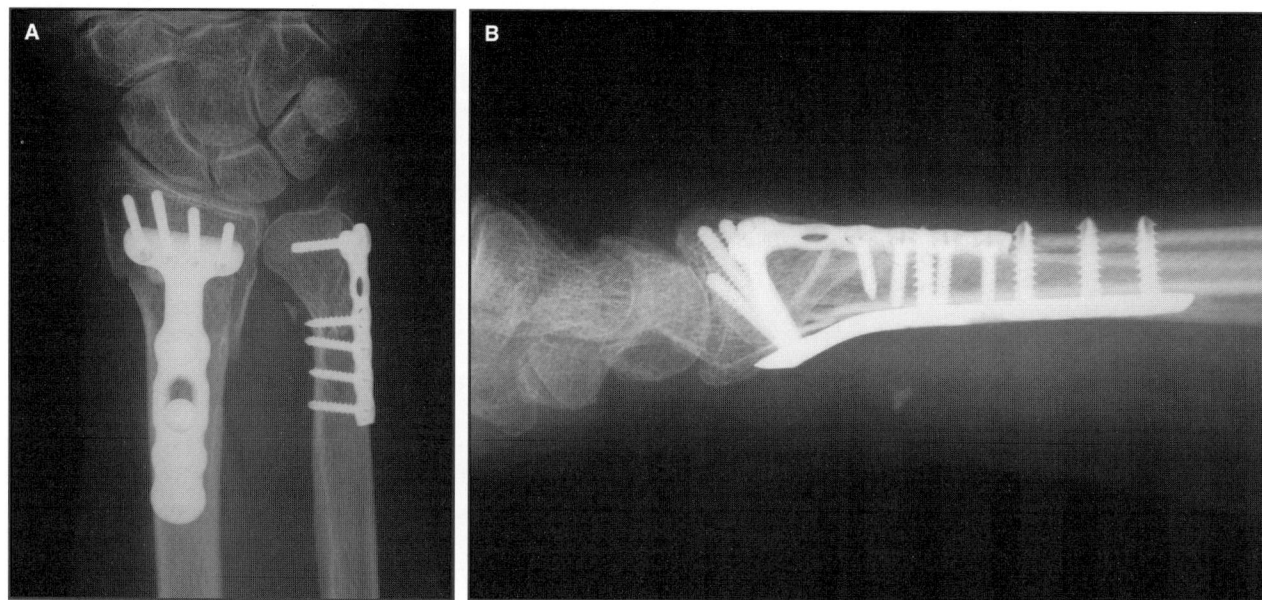

Figure 2 Initial postoperative PA **(A)** and lateral **(B)** radiographs.

decrease in wrist flexion. Additionally, increasing dorsal angulation and radial shortening can alter mechanics at the distal radioulnar joint (DRUJ), with corresponding restriction of motion.[2-4]

Other causes of wrist stiffness are considered either intra- or extra-articular. Intra-articular sources are joint arthrofibrosis and capsular and/or ligamentous shortening, thickening, and scarring. Extra-articular factors include skin and subcutaneous scarring and musculotendinous contracture or spasticity.

Treatment of contracture at the radiocarpal joint following a distal radius fracture has received little attention in the literature. Most authors describe either congenital or spastic conditions such as arthrogryposis, cerebral palsy, Dupuytren's disease, or cerebrovascular accident. Authors describing posttraumatic contracture focus principally on treatment of burn contracture.

Normal wrist motion traditionally is measured as wrist extension, wrist flexion, ulnar deviation, and radial deviation. The normal average arcs of motion have been reported by several authors.[5-7] Maximal extension averages 67°; flexion, 77°; radial deviation, 21°; and ulnar deviation, 36°.

The wrist can function well despite significant decreases in normal motion. Palmer and associates[8] evaluated functional wrist motion in 10 asymptomatic individuals during 52 standardized tasks. They reported that different tasks required specific ranges and directions of motion. Most tasks were performed in wrist extension and more than half in ulnar deviation. They concluded, based on their observation of the 52 tasks, that functional wrist motion is 5° of wrist flexion, 30° of wrist extension, 10° of radial deviation, and 15° of ulnar deviation.

Ryu and associates[7] evaluated 40 normal subjects performing tasks of personal care and hygiene, diet and food preparation, and miscellaneous activities (eg, using a hammer and screwdriver; turning a key, doorknob, and steering wheel; bringing a telephone to the ear; and writing). They reported that the entire battery of tests could be performed with 60° of extension, 54° of flexion, 40° of ulnar deviation, and 17° of radial deviation. They used these measurements to define the maximum amount of wrist motion required for daily activities. For most activities, only 70% of this motion was required: 40° of flexion and extension, 10° of radial deviation, and 30° of ulnar deviation. Wrist motion was measured with an electrogoniometer, which was found to be reliable throughout the testing. The average maximal ulnar deviation was 42.7° before testing and 42.9° after testing, whereas the hand-held measurement averaged 37.7°.

Treatment

The treatment of wrist contracture begins with prevention. The first step is the elimination of tissue edema. Edema results from injury and is characterized by protein-rich interstitial fluid. It can be controlled initially through strict elevation, compression, and finger exercises. In the short term, edema limits both active and passive motion. Without treatment, the protein-rich fluid is eventually replaced by scar tissue, typically affecting both intra- and extra-articular tissues, both at the site of injury and wherever else edema persists.

The next step is to begin ROM exercises as soon as fracture stability allows. Newer fracture fixation techniques result in sufficient initial stability to allow early ROM exercises. Both locking plates and fragment-specific fixation techniques provide rigid constructs that allow early mobilization.[9-12] When rigid fixation cannot be obtained, or when methods that require immobilization such as casts or external fixators are used, motion should be started as soon as the risk of late collapse has passed: often within 6 weeks.

With knowledge of the minimum amount of wrist flexion, extension, radial deviation, and ulnar deviation needed to perform most activities of daily living, goals can be set for the patient as soon as radiocarpal motion is allowed. These goals can then be customized based on the patient's functional demands and expectations. Initial exercises include active, active-assist, and passive ROM. These exercises can then be advanced to weighted stretches and progressive strengthening.

Patients who are slow to progress, or who plateau without achieving their goals, should begin treatment designed specifically for wrist contracture. This point usually occurs approximately 3 months after injury or surgery, when the period of inflammation and scar proliferation has passed, and scar remodeling and maturation are occurring.

The causes of wrist stiffness must be identified before beginning treatment. A detailed physical examination and standard radiographs are needed. Once the amount of stiffness is quantified by comparing motion with that in the opposite, normal wrist, potential intra- and extra-articular causes are listed. If significant residual fracture deformity exists, with more than 20° of dorsal angulation and/or 5 mm of radial shortening, a corrective osteotomy should be considered. In patients with less deformity, treatment should commence, targeting the soft-tissue components of contracture.

Nonsurgical treatment The first step in treatment of contracture is a physical therapy program designed to stretch scar tissue. The patient already should have been instructed in and compliant with standard active, active-assist, and passive ROM exercises. Significant improvements in motion are possible with the addition of dynamic and static-progressive splints.

Dynamic splinting is the use of traction devices, such as rubber bands, to alter passive ROM in the joint.[13] These splints are worn for extended periods, typically 8 to 12 hours at a time. Through prolonged, constant load, tissues respond via plastic deformation. By definition, plastic deformation is permanent in that the tissue remains in its elongated state after removal of the load. This definition is in contrast to that of elastic deformation, which occurs with rapid loading and results in only temporary tissue elongation. Dynamic splinting produces plastic deformation through creep, which is the deformation of tissue that occurs while it is placed under constant stress for an extended period of time. Tissue that is unloaded before failure occurs remains permanently lengthened as a result of its viscoplastic properties.

Static-progressive splinting and serial casting also produce plastic deformation, although through a different process: stress-relaxation. Stress-relaxation occurs when a material is held at a constant deformation. The amount of force required to maintain the deformation decreases with time as the tissue stretches by plastic deformation until equilibrium is attained.

Both methods improve motion in contracted joints.[14-17] Dynamic splints are more readily available because they can be made from materials present in most physical therapy offices. Their main disadvantage is that they must be worn for long periods to achieve lasting improvement, which may affect patient compliance. Static-progressive splints are well tolerated, effective, and require significantly less treatment time.[16]

If motion is still limited despite documented compliance with a dynamic or static-progressive splinting program, surgical treatment should be considered. The offending structure at this point is often intra-articular and consists of arthrofibrosis and capsular contracture. The surgical approach may be either open or arthroscopic but should be selected to address the underlying pathology.

Arthroscopic release Arthroscopic capsular release has been described by Verhellen and Bain.[18] They first performed cadaveric dissection and MRI to assess the

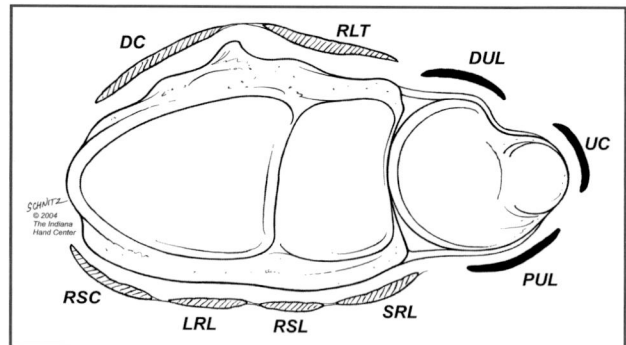

Figure 3 Cross section of the wrist with the dorsal and volar ligaments. The sectioned ligaments are cross-hatched, and the preserved ligaments are blackened. DC = dorsal capsule, RLT = dorsal radiolunotriquetral ligament, DUL = dorsal ulnolunate ligament, RSC = radioscaphocapitate ligament, LRL = long radiolunate ligament, RSL = radioscapholunate ligament, SRL = short radiolunate ligament, PUL = palmar ulnolunate ligament, UC = ulnocarpal ligament.

safety of the procedure by calculating the distance of neurovascular structures from the joint capsule. The median nerve averaged 6.9 mm, the ulnar nerve 6.7 mm, and the radial artery 5.2 mm from the volar wrist capsule. Arthroscopic release was then performed in two patients who gained an average of 30° of flexion and 40° of extension.

The technique is performed with a standard arthroscopic tower and 10 lb of traction. The 3-4 and 6-R portals are created, and the joint is débrided of adhesions and synovitis. The volar capsule is divided, with the arthroscope in the 3-4 portal and a hooked electrocautery probe in the 6-R portal. The electrocautery probe is advanced radially as far as possible, and the volar capsule is divided to the ulnar border of the radius, leaving the ulnotriquetral and ulnolunate ligaments intact. The release includes the radioscaphocapitate, long radiolunate, radioscapholunate, and short radiolunate ligaments and is complete when extracarpal fat and the flexor carpi radialis tendon are visualized.[18] The dorsal release is performed with the electrocautery probe placed in the 1-2 portal, and the capsule is divided beginning at the sigmoid notch and continuing to the 1-2 portal. This procedure releases the dorsal radiocarpal ligament but leaves the dorsal ulnar ligament complex intact (**Figure 3**).

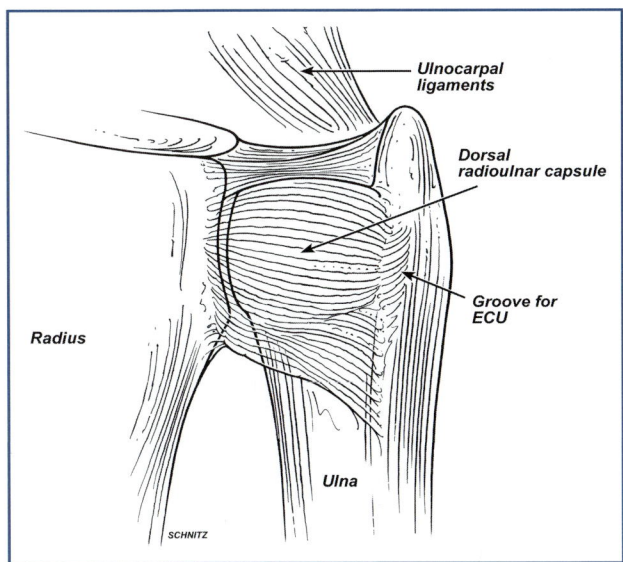

Figure 4 Anatomy of dorsal radiocarpal joint. Release is performed along the margin of the distal radius. ECU = extensor carpi ulnaris.

Despite release of the important volar ligamentous support of the carpus, ulnar translation did not develop in either of Verhellen and Bain's[18] patients. They based their approach on the work of Viegas and associates[19] who reported that either the palmar ulnolunate or the dorsal ulnolunate ligament complex alone can prevent ulnar translation. At this time, however, caution is warranted. With only two cases reported in the literature and limited follow-up evaluation, I preserve the volar ligaments, if at all possible.

Open techniques Open release is indicated in patients with combined intra- and extra-articular sources of contracture, when the patient has other pathology that requires treatment, or when arthroscopy is not technically feasible. Open approaches may be dorsal, volar, or combined as described by Watson and Weinzweig.[20] Either transverse or longitudinal incisions may be used.

In the dorsal approach (**Figure 4**), the capsule is divided along the radiocarpal joint. Intra-articular scar is excised and wrist motion checked. If the lunate lifts off of the radius with wrist flexion and a resulting loss of articular congruency, or if a lack of wrist extension persists, a volar approach is recommended to release the volar scar.

The volar approach may be performed through either a transverse or longitudinal incision. Retraction of the flexor tendons and median nerve is facilitated by releasing the transverse carpal ligament along its ulnar border. The deep scar, which usually lies superficial to the intrinsic radiocarpal ligaments, is then excised. The underlying ligaments run obliquely, and an attempt should be made to preserve them, if possible.

Full active, active-assist, and passive ROM is begun on postoperative day 1. The bulky, compressive postoperative dressing is debulked, and resting wrist extension and/or flexion splints may be used between exercise sessions to maintain the improvements obtained at surgery. Postoperative pain is controlled by indwelling catheters that release bupivacaine into the surgical site over the first 3 to 5 days and by scheduled doses of oral analgesics and anti-inflammatory medication.

Management and Outcome Summary

At 6-week follow-up, the patient had achieved only modest improvements in motion with a standard physical therapy program. Guided physical therapy was continued, and dynamic splinting was added to improve wrist flexion. Use of the interval splint was discontinued. The patient was encouraged to use the arm for more daily activities. Additionally, a gentle, progressive strengthening program was begun.

Four months postoperatively, excellent improvements in flexion and extension were achieved. Wrist extension was 70° and flexion 50°. Sensibility continued to be normal. The patient had no pain at rest or with light activities and only mild pain with heavy use. However, the patient continued to have significantly restricted forearm pronation and supination.

RADIOULNAR STIFFNESS AND CONTRACTURE
Case Presentation

Four months postoperatively, the same patient reported difficulty with daily activities and playing golf. He stated that it was hard for him to turn keys, open doors, and open jars. Radiographs showed healing of

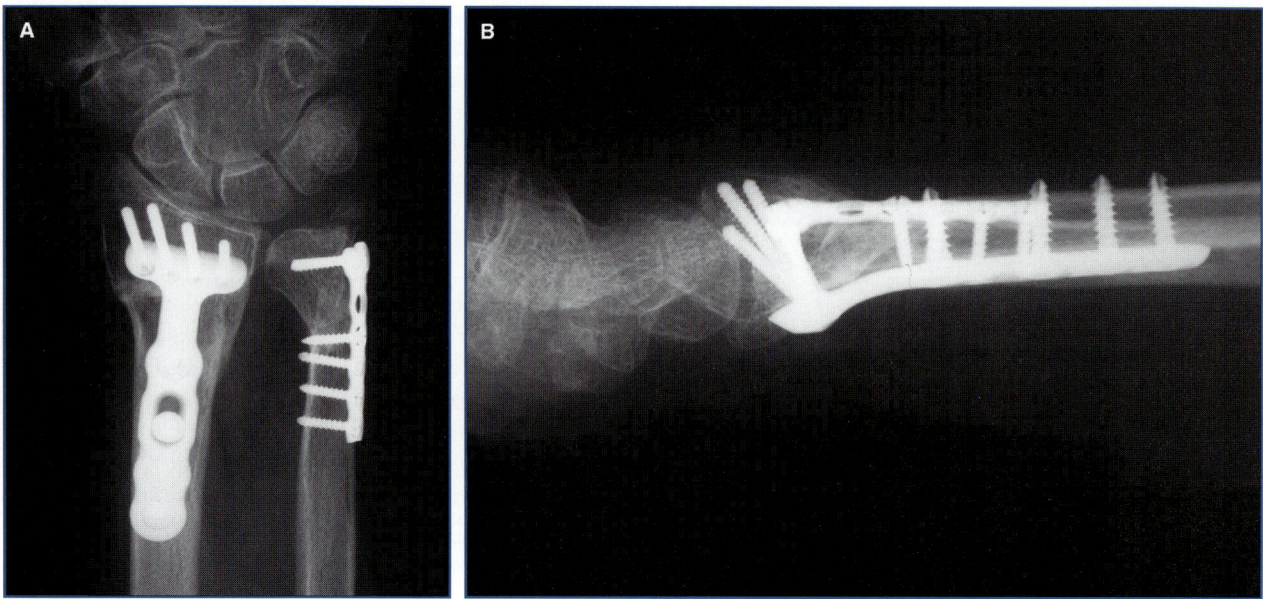

Figure 5 PA **(A)** and lateral **(B)** radiographs at 4 months after surgery.

the distal radius and ulnar neck fractures in acceptable alignment, but with an ulnar styloid nonunion (**Figure 5**). Supination was limited to 40° and pronation was 65°. The patient was frustrated.

Discussion
Clinical Assessment

Loss of pronation and supination can be disabling to patients in their work, hobbies, and everyday activities, even when they have functional radiocarpal motion. In most patients, pronation is the principal direction of motion used for grasping, eating, and writing. Loss of pronation is well compensated for by shoulder abduction. Supination is necessary for tasks such as personal hygiene, opening door handles, and taking change but is poorly compensated for by shoulder function. Patients typically lose functional supination rather than pronation after a distal radius fracture.

In a study of functional elbow motion, Morrey and associates[21] reported that the normal arc of pronosupination is 170°, with functional motion as 50° of pronation and 50° of supination. Limited supination and pronation to an arc of 30° to 50° in each direction

prevented their patients from performing 5 of 15 standard tasks, whereas patients with a total arc of 30° of pronosupination could perform only six tasks. They also reported that a 100° arc of motion allowed patients to perform all 15 tasks without functional limitation or modification of behavior.

Causes of DRUJ stiffness may be intrinsic to the joint or secondary to malunion. Intra-articular causes include posttraumatic osteoarthritis from residual articular incongruity, arthrofibrosis, and capsular contracture. Distal radial malunion plays a significant role in limiting motion at the DRUJ. Kihara and associates[4] reported that progressive dorsal angulation of the distal radius increases tightness of the interosseous membrane and DRUJ incongruency, with compensatory decreases in maximum pronation and supination. A change of more than 30° of dorsal angulation (more than 20° of dorsal tilt measured radiographically) resulted in statistically significant limitations of supination and pronation, whereas a change of 20° or more resulted in increasing incongruency of the DRUJ. Radial shortening of 5 to 6 mm increases tension in the triangular fibrocartilage complex (TFCC) and limits pronation and supination.[3,22]

Knowledge of the complex anatomy of the DRUJ is

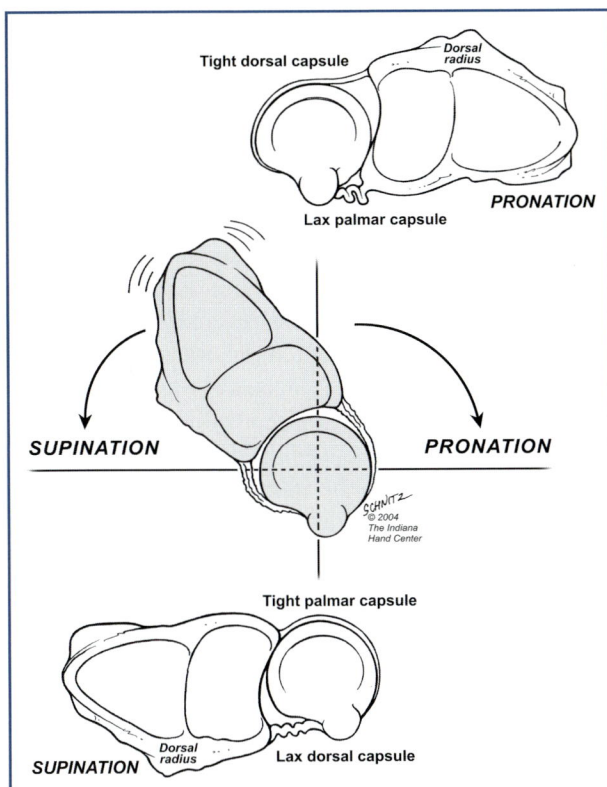

Figure 6 Detail of the dorsal and palmar radioulnar ligaments. In supination, the volar capsule is draped over the ulnar head and taut, wheras the dorsal capsule relaxes. As the radius rotates around the fixed ulna into pronation, the volar capsule becomes patulous, whereas the dorsal capsule tightens.

crucial to an understanding of the etiology of DRUJ contracture. The capsule of the DRUJ is tripartite, with dorsal, proximal, and volar components.[23] Distally, the TFCC forms the roof of the joint and is critical for joint stability. The TFCC comprises the dorsal and volar radioulnar ligaments, the central avascular articular disk, the disk-carpal ligaments, the volar sheath of the extensor carpi ulnaris tendon, and the ulnocarpal meniscal homolog. The dorsal and volar radioulnar ligaments provide the main stability to the DRUJ. The dorsal radioulnar ligament becomes taut with the joint in full pronation, and the volar radioulnar ligament tightens with the joint in full supination (**Figure 6**).[24-26] Both ligaments provide stability in all positions of forearm rotation; however,

the dorsal ligament provides greater restraint to translation with the DRUJ in pronation, and the volar ligament provides greater restraint in supination.[24]

The capsular components of the DRUJ are distinct. The thin volar leaf is patulous, having a redundant oblique fold that accommodates the ulnar head during forearm supination. The dorsal leaf has less redundancy, is slightly thinner, and tightens with forearm pronation.[23] Supination contracture occurs more commonly than pronation contracture because of these differences. Both the dorsal and volar capsules can become thickened as a result of posttraumatic fibrosis; however, as the volar capsule loses its redundant fold, it can no longer accommodate the ulnar head in supination.

Treatment

Treatment of DRUJ contracture, like that for radiocarpal contracture, begins with aggressive edema control, and early initiation of motion is paramount, regardless of how the fracture was treated. Once the fracture is sufficiently stable to allow forearm rotation, the patient should be instructed in active supination and pronation exercises. Goals should be set for the patient, with a minimum range of 50° of both pronation and supination.

Nonsurgical treatment Patients who have an established or impending DRUJ contracture without significant radial malunion, DRUJ articular incongruity, or DRUJ arthrosis and in whom conventional physical therapy has failed require further treatment. As in treatment for radiocarpal stiffness, the next phase after conventional physical therapy is the addition of dynamic or static-progressive splints.

Dynamic splinting has been shown to be effective. In a study of 15 patients with DRUJ contracture, Shah and associates[27] were able to increase the average arc of motion by 52%. Their inclusion criteria consisted of an acceptably healed distal radius fracture (≤ 20° of dorsal tilt and ≤ 5 mm of ulnar variance) and failure to obtain functional pronosupination despite conventional hand therapy for an average of 8 weeks. Patients wore the splint for 6 hours per day if either pronation or supination contractures were being treated, or 12 hours for both pronation and supination contractures. Average forearm rotation before

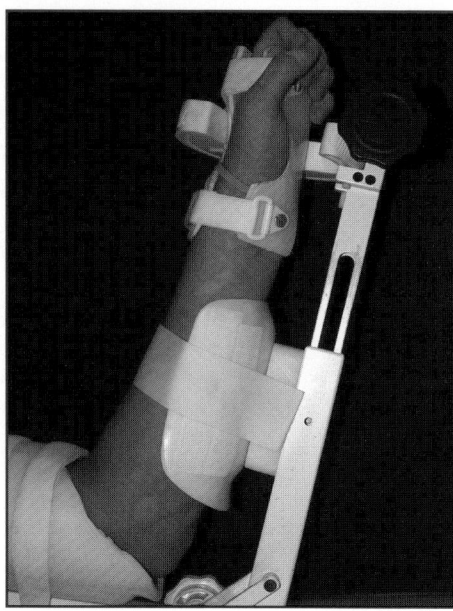

Figure 7 Patient using a static-progressive splint in full pronation.

splinting was 83° and increased 126° after an average of 11 weeks of treatment.

Static-progressive splinting also can be used for DRUJ contracture (**Figure 7**). This type of splint localizes the stretching force at the DRUJ. It can correct to 120° of supination and 100° of pronation. It is worn for 30 minute sessions, with each session targeted to either pronation or supination. Total treatment consists of up to three sessions daily for either pronation or supination, or six sessions for both.

Silhouette capsulectomy Indications for surgery are relative and depend on the patient's functional needs. Achieving a 100° arc of pronosupination allows patients to resume most activities. When the arc of motion precludes normal occupational and lifestyle requirements, and nonsurgical treatment lasting more than 6 months has failed, including dynamic or static-progressive splinting, surgical treatment is warranted.

The concept of silhouette capsulectomy, originally described by Kleinman and Graham[23] and later by Kleinman,[28] is to excise the contracted capsule of the DRUJ while preserving the necessary ligamentous support of the joint. The approach is tailored to the patient's functional limitations. In patients with limited forearm pronation, the contracted dorsal capsule needs to be excised. With loss of supination, it is the scarred volar capsule that limits motion. In either case, the dorsal and volar radioulnar ligaments, as well as the inferior aspect of the capsule, are preserved because they do not restrict motion.

Most patients with functional loss of forearm rotation have restricted supination. The approach to the volar capsule of the DRUJ is through the interval between the ulnar neurovascular bundle and the flexor carpi ulnaris tendon. Gentle retraction exposes the palmar radioulnar ligament and palmar capsule of the DRUJ. The capsule is first incised along its distal margin, just proximal to the palmar radioulnar ligament, from ulnar to radial. Care is taken to protect the ligament by identifying the interval between the ulnar pole and the TFCC; identification is facilitated by placing a hypodermic needle into the interval. The ligament is then resected along its radial margin to the proximal edge of the sigmoid notch. The dissection is continued ulnarly up to the metaphysis of the distal ulna. Finally, the ulnar attachment is released along the margin of the articular surface of the ulnar head. In this manner, the silhouette of the ulnar head on the volar capsule is excised. Once the capsule has been removed, any intra-articular adhesions can be freed with a periosteal elevator.[23,28]

In patients with restricted forearm pronation, the dorsal DRUJ capsule is excised (**Figure 8**). The approach is through a longitudinal or transverse skin incision. The fifth dorsal compartment is incised, and the extensor digiti quinti retracted. The floor of the fifth dorsal compartment directly overlies and is distinct from the underlying dorsal DRUJ capsule. It may be separated and protected; however, it is technically easier to excise it along with the capsule. The capsular incision is begun distally, just proximal to the dorsal radioulnar ligament. As with the volar capsulectomy, care must be taken to protect the ligament from iatrogenic injury. The capsule is released along its radial attachment to the proximal margin of the sigmoid notch. The silhouette of the ulnar head is then traced medially to the metaphysis of the ulna and, finally, detached from its ulnar insertion. Intra-articular adhesions are then excised.[23,28]

Postoperatively, a bulky short arm dressing is placed, and ROM exercises are begun as soon as possible. Ideally, the surgery is performed under regional

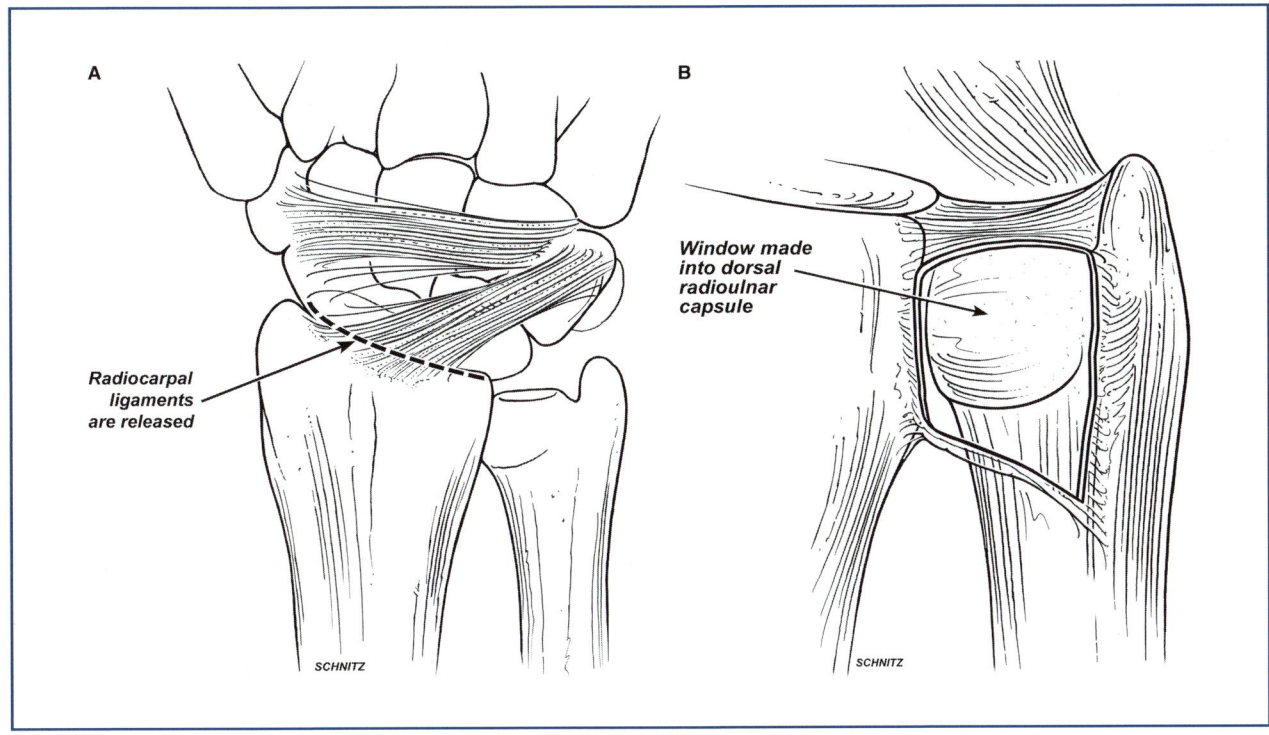

Figure 8 A, Dorsal view of the DRUJ. The capsule attaches to the radial margin, ulnar neck, and proximal fibers of the TFCC. Capsular tissue is thickened and stiff in the presence of a DRUJ contracture. **B,** The window of the dorsal capsule has been excised, and the radioulnar ligament and inferior capsule have been preserved. The volar procedure is identical.

anesthesia, and the patient is instructed in passive forearm supination and pronation exercises to begin while the arm is numb. Once motor recovery begins, active and active-assist exercises are added. As with all capsulectomy procedures, patient compliance is paramount to a successful result. By following a guided rehabilitation program, motivated patients can be expected to maintain the improvements obtained at surgery.[23]

Management and Outcome Summary

Despite aggressive physical therapy, including dynamic splinting and weighted stretches, the patient continued to have forearm stiffness that interfered with his activities, particularly golf. His supination continued to be limited to 40° and pronation to 65°.

DRUJ capsulectomy was recommended and performed 6 months after his initial surgery.

With the patient under axillary block anesthesia, a volar DRUJ silhouette capsulectomy was performed as previously described. Passive intraoperative supination was 85° without rebound, although pronation continued to be limited. A dorsal approach was performed next, and the dorsal DRUJ capsule excised, with resultant passive pronation of 90°.

The patient continued aggressive physical therapy on the day after surgery. Initially, he was only able to maintain 65° of pronation and supination because of pain and swelling. Over the next 5 weeks, he continued physical therapy and made steady progress. At his 6-week follow-up, pronation was 75° and supination 70°. The patient was pleased with these improvements and was placed on a home exercise program for continued active motion, passive stretching, and progressive strengthening.

REFERENCES

1. Knirk JL, Jupiter JB: Intra-articular fractures of the distal end of the radius in young adults. *J Bone Joint Surg Am* 1986;68:647-659.

2. Fernandez DL: Correction of post-traumatic wrist deformity in adults by osteotomy, bone-grafting, and internal fixation. *J Bone Joint Surg Am* 1982;64:1164-1178.

3. Adams BD: Effects of radial deformity on distal radioulnar joint mechanics. *J Hand Surg [Am]* 1993;18:492-498.

4. Kihara H, Palmer AK, Werner FW, Short WH, Fortino MD: The effect of dorsally angulated distal radius fractures on distal radioulnar joint congruency and forearm rotation. *J Hand Surg [Am]* 1996;21:40-47.

5. Brumfield RH Jr, Nickel VL, Nickel E: Joint motion in wrist flexion and extension. *South Med J* 1966;59:909-910.

6. Boone DC, Azen SP: Normal range of motion of joints in male subjects. *J Bone Joint Surg Am* 1979; 61:756-759.

7. Ryu JY, Cooney WP III, Askew LJ, An KN, Chao EY: Functional ranges of motion of the wrist joint. *J Hand Surg [Am]* 1991;16:409-419.

8. Palmer AK, Werner FW, Murphy D, Glisson R: Functional wrist motion: A biomechanical study. *J Hand Surg [Am]* 1985;10:39-46.

9. Konrath GA, Bahler S: Open reduction and internal fixation of unstable distal radius fractures: Results using the trimed fixation system. *J Orthop Trauma* 2002;16:578-585.

10. Swigart CR, Wolfe SW: Limited incision open techniques for distal radius fracture management. *Orthop Clin North Am* 2001;32:317-327.

11. Orbay JL: The treatment of unstable distal radius fractures with volar fixation. *Hand Surg* 2000;5:103-112.

12. Orbay JL, Fernandez DL: Volar fixation for dorsally displaced fractures of the distal radius: A preliminary report. *J Hand Surg [Am]* 2002;27:205-215.

13. Fessm EE, Philips CA: *Hand Splinting: Principles and Methods.* St Louis, MO, Mosby, 1987, p 74.

14. Prosser R: Splinting in the management of proximal interphalangeal joint flexion contracture. *J Hand Ther* 1996;9:378-386.

15. Scheker LR, Chesher SP, Netscher DT, Julliard KN, O'Neill WL: Functional results of dynamic splinting after transmetacarpal, wrist, and distal forearm replantation. *J Hand Surg [Br]* 1995;20:584-590.

16. Bonutti PM, Windau JE, Ables BA, Miller BG: Static progressive stretch to reestablish elbow range of motion. *Clin Orthop* 1994;303:128-134.

17. Duncan RM: Basic principles of splinting the hand. *Phys Therapy* 1989;69:1104-1116.

18. Verhellen R, Bain GI: Arthroscopic capsular release for contracture of the wrist: A new technique. *Arthroscopy* 2000;16:106-110.

19. Viegas SF, Patterson RM, Ward K: Extrinsic wrist ligaments in the pathomechanics of ulnar translation instability. *J Hand Surg [Am]* 1995;20:312-318.

20. Watson HK, Weinzweig J: Stiff joints, in Green DP, Hotchkiss RN, Pederson WC (eds): *Green's Operative Hand* Surgery. New York, NY, Churchill Livingstone, 1999, p 559.

21. Morrey BF, Askew LJ, Chao EY: A biomechanical study of normal functional elbow motion. *J Bone Joint Surg Am* 1981;63:872-877.

22. Jupiter JB, Masem M: Reconstruction of post-traumatic deformity of the distal radius and ulna. *Hand Clin* 1988;4:377-390.

23. Kleinman WB, Graham TJ: The distal radioulnar joint capsule: Clinical anatomy and role in post-traumatic limitation of forearm rotation. *J Hand Surg [Am]* 1998; 23:588-599.

24. Ward LD, Ambrose CG, Masson MV, Levaro F: The role of the distal radioulnar ligaments, interosseous membrane, and joint capsule in distal radioulnar joint stability. *J Hand Surg [Am]* 2000;25:341-351.

25. Schuind F, An KN, Berglund L, et al: The distal radioulnar ligaments: A biomechanical study. *J Hand Surg [Am]* 1991;16:1106-1114.

26. Hagert CG: Distal radius fracture and the distal radioulnar joint: Anatomical considerations. *Handchir Mikrochir Plast Chir* 1994;26:22-26.

27. Shah MA, Lopez JK, Escalante AS, Green DP: Dynamic splinting of forearm rotational contracture after distal radius fracture. *J Hand Surg [Am]* 2002;27:456-463.

28. Kleinman WB: DRUJ contracture release. *Tech Hand Upper Extremity Surg* 1999;3:1-22.

Chapter 5

NEUROLOGIC COMPLICATIONS

F. Thomas D. Kaplan, MD

PRESENTATION

A 57-year-old right-handed woman sustained a displaced intra-articular distal radius fracture and an ulnar styloid fracture in the left wrist in a fall while roller skating. She also had a 3-mm laceration on the ulnar aspect of her wrist. She was initially treated with urgent surgical repair, including placement of an external fixator and percutaneous pins. Approximately 1 week after surgery, the patient reported increasing pain that was poorly controlled with narcotic analgesics. Radiographs taken on postoperative day 11 demonstrated residual articular incongruity and significant radiocarpal distraction (**Figure 1**). The initial treating physician referred her for pain management 5 weeks after surgery, and she presented for a second opinion.

At the time of second-opinion evaluation, 5.5 weeks after surgery, the patient reported constant burning and pain in her wrist and fingers. She described a tingling sensation in all fingers, reporting that they felt as if they were "on fire." Physical examination revealed mild erythema over her dorsal and ulnar wrist. Her fingers were diffusely swollen, and she had minimal motion at the metacarpophalangeal and interphalangeal joints (**Figure 2**). Her external fixator pin and Kirschner wire (K-wire) sites were clean and dry. The hand and fingers were warm, sweaty, and diffusely hypersensitive. She also had ipsilateral shoulder stiffness with forward elevation limited to 100° and external rotation to 30°. Radiographs showed progressive fracture consolidation, ulnar styloid nonunion, and persistent increased radiocarpal distraction (**Figure 3**).

DISCUSSION

Patients who present with severe, diffuse pain and hypersensitivity following treatment of a distal radius fracture must be carefully evaluated for potential cause of these symptoms, including infection, nonunion, malunion, hardware migration, tendon inflammation or rupture, and nerve compression or injury. When, after careful clinical examination, no specific etiology can be found, reflex sympathetic dystrophy (RSD) is frequently diagnosed. RSD is just one of several terms for this condition. Other terms, often used interchangeably, include Sudek's atrophy, algodystrophy, shoulder-hand syndrome, causalgia, and sympathetically mediated pain (SMP). The term RSD itself is confusing because it implies that the sympathetic nervous system is responsible for the syndrome

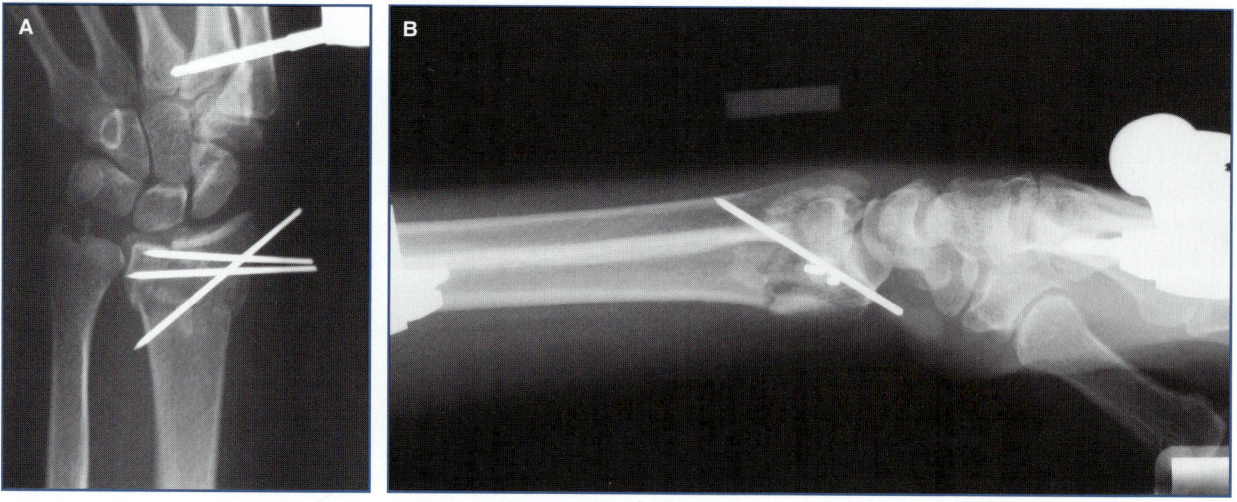

Figure 1 PA **(A)** and lateral **(B)** radiographs 11 days after surgery. Note the distracted radiocarpal space.

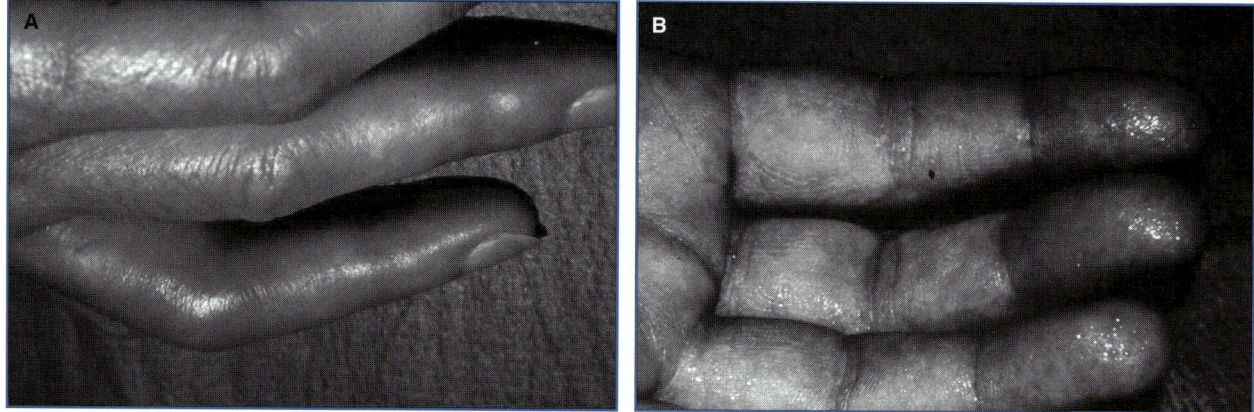

Figure 2 Clinical photographs obtained 5.5 weeks postoperatively show rubor and edema on the dorsal view **(A)** and rubor, edema, and sweating on the palmar view **(B)**.

and that it starts as a reflex, which, by definition, occurs automatically in response to a stimulus.

Because of the difficulty in accurately applying the diagnosis of RSD and poor attempts to standardize research, the International Association for the Study of Pain (IASP) proposed new terminology in 1994.[1] Chronic regional pain syndrome (CRPS) type I replaces RSD, and CRPS type II replaces causalgia. Although both terms describe identical clinical presentations, type II is used when the patient has an identifiable, discrete nerve lesion, whereas type I is used for patients who have no specific nerve injury.[1]

The diagnostic criteria proposed for CRPS consist of the following: (1) a syndrome that develops following an initiating noxious event or cause of immobilization (type I) or that develops after a discrete nerve injury (type II); (2) spontaneous pain, allodynia (painful response to nonpainful stimuli), or hyperalgesia (increased response to painful stimuli) that is not limited to the territory of a single peripheral nerve and is disproportionate to the initiating injury; (3) evidence at some point of edema, changes in skin blood flow, or abnormal sudomotor activity in the region of pain; and (4) no evidence of another condition that would

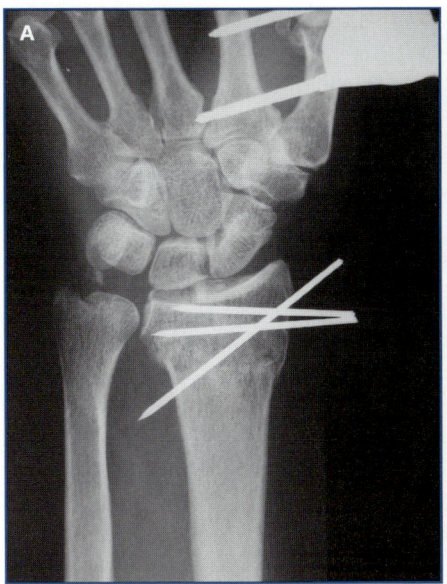
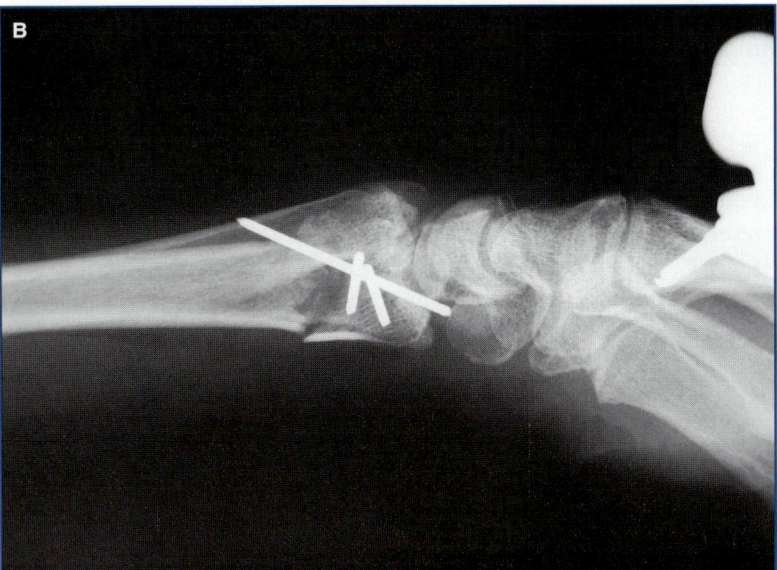

Figure 3 PA **(A)** and lateral **(B)** radiographs 5.5 weeks after surgery.

TABLE 1 Proposed Diagnostic Criteria for CRPS

Pain	**Reported Symptom***	**Displayed Symptom†**
Continuing; disproportionate to any inciting event	Sensory	Sensory
	Hyperesthesia	Hyperalgesia (to pinprick)
		Allodynia (to light touch)
	Vasomotor	Vasomotor
	Temperature asymmetry	Temperature asymmetry
	Skin color changes	Skin color changes
	Skin color asymmetry	Skin color asymmetry
	Sudomotor/edema	Sudomotor/edema
	Edema	Edema
	Sweating changes	Sweating changes
	Sweating asymmetry	Sweating asymmetry
	Motor/trophic	Motor/trophic
	Decreased range of motion	Decreased range of motion
	Motor dysfunction (weakness, tremor, dystonia)	Motor dysfunction (weakness, tremor, dystonia)
	Trophic changes (hair, nail, skin)	Trophic changes (hair, nail, skin)

*Must report at least one symptom in each category
† Must display at least one symptom in each category

account for the degree and nature of pain and dysfunction. These criteria have not been fully validated, and, in fact, a modification has been proposed to improve the diagnostic accuracy.[2,3] The proposed criteria are detailed in **Table 1**.

The creation of standardized diagnostic criteria should improve both the ability to diagnose patients and the ability to study this confusing condition. Despite these new criteria, the diagnosis of CRPS type I continues to be difficult as a result of the myriad presentations of the condition and the lack of a gold standard diagnostic test.

CRPS Type I

The incidence of CRPS type I following distal radius fractures has been reported to range from less than 2% to 37%.[4,5] The wide range is thought to be secondary to the variability of criteria used to define the disease and of the effort clinicians make to look for the condition.

Natural History

The natural history of CRPS type I is unknown. Traditionally, it is believed to progress through three phases: acute, dystrophic, and atrophic. The acute phase, from onset to 3 months, is characterized by symptoms of constant burning, allodynia, hyperalgesia, edema, and sudomotor changes. In the dystrophic stage, 3 to 9 months after onset, there is persistent pain, stiffness, loss of skin creases and hair, and a change from redness to cyanosis in the extremity. Patients in the atrophic stage, 9 to 18 months following injury, typically have a cool, pale, dry limb, fixed contractures, and severe osteopenia. This progression has not been supported by prospective studies, although several authors suggest that the condition does not progress but rather tends to remain stable or improve over time.[6-8] Harden and associates[3] proposed that the characteristics of multiple, distinct subtypes of the disorder account for the differences previously attributed to clinical stages.

Every patient who fractures his or her distal radius may be at risk for CRPS type I. Therefore, this diagnosis must be considered in all patients who report pain more severe than normally would be expected. Because the diagnosis is clinical, it cannot be confirmed with objective testing, even though a number of diagnostic tests may be helpful in supporting the clinical impression. No test has achieved the status of gold standard because of poor or inconsistent sensitivity and specificity. In fact, a gold standard test is unlikely until standardized diagnostic criteria are identified, accepted, and validated.

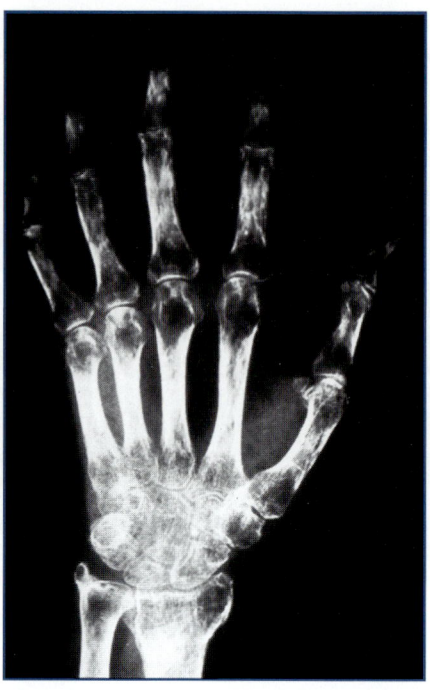

Figure 4 Radiograph of a right hand with a healed distal radius fracture. Note the marked periarticular osteopenia.

Imaging Studies

Plain radiographs may show osteopenia in the affected limb, beginning in a patchy periarticular pattern and progressing to a more diffuse ground-glass appearance[9] (**Figure 4**). A three-phase bone scan may confirm the diagnosis of CRPS type I. A positive scan typically shows diffusely increased uptake in the third phase, in a periarticular pattern involving multiple joints (**Figure 5**). However, the accuracy of the three-phase bone scan for this condition remains in question. In a review of studies reporting the sensitivity, specificity, positive predictive value, and negative predictive value of the three-phase bone scan, Lee and Weeks[10] reported that the accuracy of the test varied widely. The best correlation between clinical diagnosis and the bone scan (sensitivity of approximately 50%) occurred with testing within 20 to 26 weeks of the onset of disease.[10] Other conditions with similar findings on three-phase bone scan include immobilization, denervation, stroke, cellulitis, and venous, arterial, and/or lymphatic obstruction. MRI may show

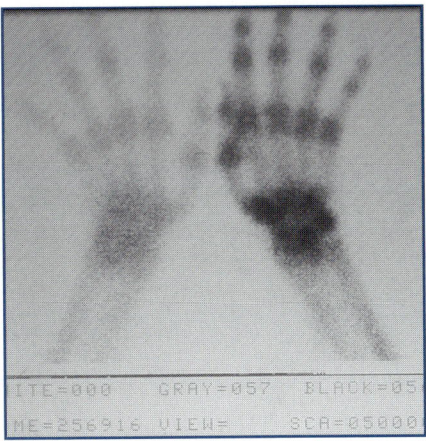

Figure 5 Three-phase bone scan demonstrating increased periarticular uptake in the right wrist and hand.

periarticular marrow edema, synovial effusion, and soft-tissue thickening but has not been found to be diagnostic.

Diagnostic Studies

The sympathetic nervous system may or may not be involved in CRPS type I. The presence of SMP can be confirmed with pain relief following stellate (cervicothoracic) ganglion block. However, because of the invasive nature and associated risks of these blocks, identifying patients who will benefit from them before they are administered is preferred. Three tests can be used to help achieve this goal: (1) the phentolamine infusion test, (2) resting sweat output test, and (3) the quantitative sudomotor axon reflex test. With the phentolamine test, α-adrenergic receptors are nonspecifically blocked, preventing the transmission of sympathetic efferent pathways at the synapse. Patients are prevented from seeing when the infusion begins; thus, a significant reduction in pain coincident with administration of phentolamine implies a significant contribution of SMP.[11] The resting sweat output test measures the sweat output of nonstimulated skin in the affected and normal extremity, whereas the quantitative sudomotor axon reflex test measures the sweat response after application of an electric current and

acetylcholine. In both of these latter tests, an abnormal result is an increased amount of sweat in the affected limb.[9]

Treatment of CRPS Type I

Many treatments have been described for CRPS type I with varying degrees of success, including physical and occupational therapy, pharmacologic agents, behavioral modification and psychotherapy, and neuromodulation through chemical sympathetic block or surgical sympathectomy. Treatment recommendations have been refined over the past decade as physicians learned more about this condition. Traditional therapies aimed solely at blocking the sympathetic nervous system, including stellate ganglion blocks and surgical sympathectomy, have yielded to more multidisciplinary approaches (**Figure 6**).

In a consensus statement on treatment of CRPS types I and II, Stanton-Hicks and associates[12] emphasized the importance of establishing rapport and a therapeutic alliance with the patient, as well as motivation, mobilization, and desensitization. Establishing rapport with patients and encouraging them to become active participants in treatment becomes more difficult the longer they have the condition. When patients are seen within the first few months of the onset of symptoms, psychological changes usually have not occurred. They expect to get well at this point, and referral to counseling is not needed. Patients with pain lasting longer than 6 months, however, often are depressed, anxious, and have disturbed sleeping patterns. These patients often benefit from formal counseling and antidepressant medication.

The cornerstone of treatment is the rehabilitation of the affected limb through edema control, mobilization, desensitization, and, ultimately, strengthening. Formal physical therapy is beneficial and initially helps the patient to avoid or overcome movement phobia. Through early desensitization and pain control, patients can more fully participate in their recovery. Stress loading with a scrubbing and carrying program aids desensitization and promotes active movement. Increased tolerance leads to improved gains in motion, decreased edema, and, ultimately, improved functional recovery.

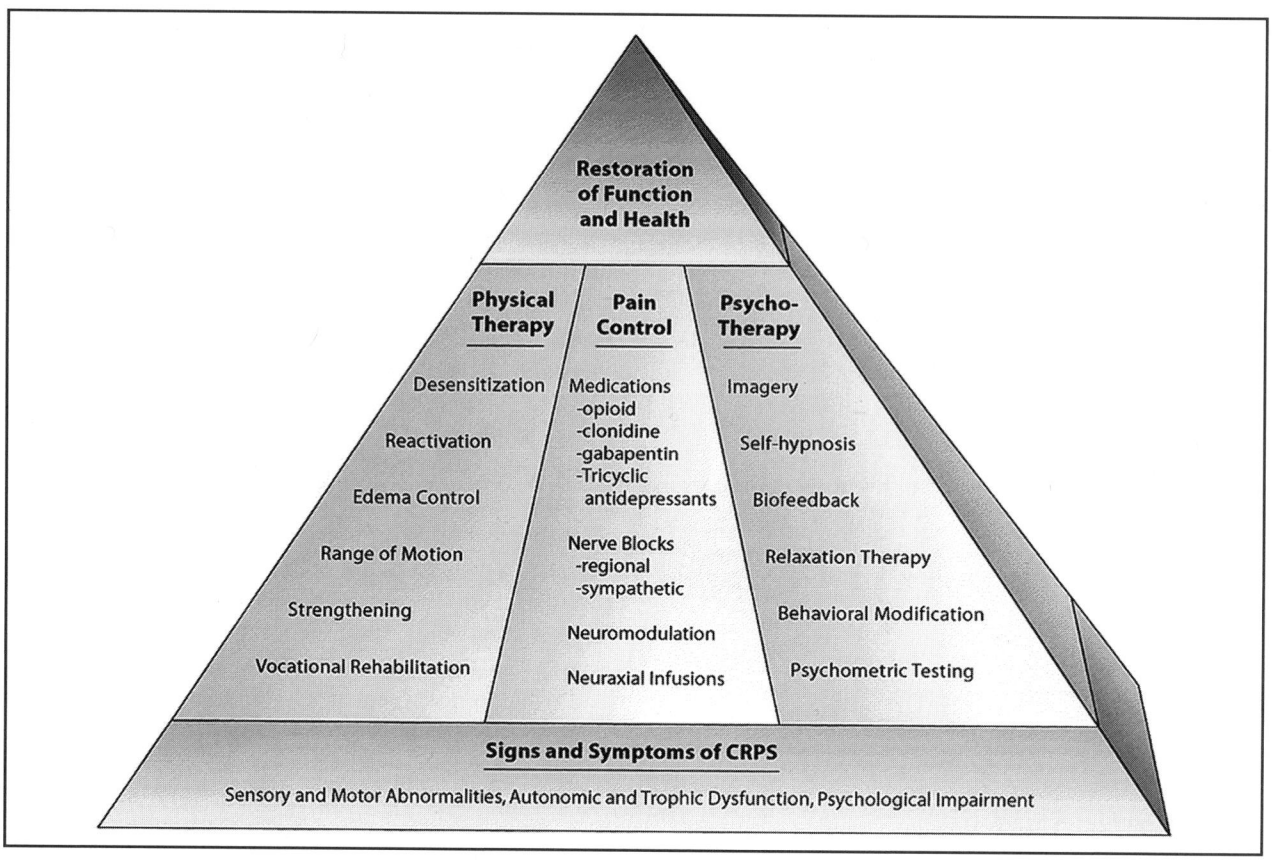

Figure 6 Multidisciplinary approach to treatment of CRPS type I. Treatment involves all necessary pharmacologic and interventional modalities necessary to control symptoms and allow functional recovery. (Reproduced with permission from Raja SN, Grabow TS: Complex regional pain syndrome I (reflex sympathetic dystrophy). *Anesthesiology* 2002;96:1254-1260.)

Pharmacologic Treatment

The addition of pharmacologic agents usually is required to reduce pain and sensitivity before patients are able to effectively participate in their recovery. These agents, however, should be considered only as a means to an end. None can stop or reverse the syndrome; rather, they work to diminish symptoms. Continual reevaluation of the patient's medication regimen is critical as treatment continues. If recovery plateaus or increased pain prevents rehabilitation, the medication profile should be reviewed and changes or additions made as appropriate. Many different agents have been used, but few have the support of randomized trials.

First-line analgesics include nonsteroidal anti-inflammatory drugs (NSAIDs), but these frequently fail to fully relieve the pain associated with CRPS type I, although they may prove useful as adjuncts. If therapeutic levels of one agent fail to provide adequate pain control, an agent from a different NSAID class should be tried. Opioid use is controversial in patients with neuropathic pain; therefore, other agents should be tried first. Opioid use in patients with a history of chemical dependence is relatively contraindicated, but in selected patients, opioids may prove to be beneficial.

Tricyclic antidepressants have been effective in treating neuropathic pain, with the best evidence for amitriptyline and imipramine. At least one in three patients will achieve at least 50% pain relief.[9] The mechanism of action is unknown, although it appears to be specific to the tricyclic antidepressants; the selective serotonin reuptake inhibitors have not been shown to be more effective than placebo in nondepressed patients with neuropathic pain.

Anticonvulsants also have been shown, through randomized clinical trials, to be effective in the treatment of neuropathic pain. Gabapentin, in doses as high as 3,600 mg/day, is effective in relieving pain associated with postherpetic neuralgia and diabetic neuropathy. Its use for CRPS (US Food and Drug Administration off-label indication) is supported only in case series.[9]

Two other medications that have been shown to be effective are corticosteroids and bisphosphonates. Corticosteroids are recommended in early phases of CRPS, especially in patients who present with edema, warmth, and rubor.[12] Their use is supported by few studies, which are limited by small sample size and single-blinded design.[9] The efficacy of bisphosphonates is also based on limited study. A single randomized controlled trial involving 20 patients treated with alendronate showed improvements in pain, motion, tenderness, and swelling within 2 weeks of treatment.[13] After 1 year, 16 patients were available for follow-up; of these, only 9 were considered to be in remission.

Other medications reported to be effective in the treatment of CRPS include capsaicin, calcium channel blockers, N-methyl-D-aspartate-receptor antagonists, topical clonidine, topical dimethyl sulfoxide, calcitonin, and intravenous ketanserin. At this time, these agents have only limited support in the literature as a result of either poor study design or conflicting results.[14]

Nerve Blocks

Sympathetic blockade through chemical or surgical means has long been promoted for the treatment of CRPS type I. The initial belief that CRPS type I was characterized by overactivity of the sympathetic nervous system led to techniques to block its function. These techniques include local anesthetic block of the sympathetic chain, intravenous guanethidine, intravenous phentolamine, and surgical sympathectomy. Despite a long history of regional sympathetic blockades,

few randomized controlled studies support their efficacy.

Intravenous guanethidine provides a regional sympathetic blockade by inhibiting the presynaptic release and reuptake of norepinephrine from postganglionic sympathetic nerve endings. Reports of its efficacy are based on case series; however, three double-blinded randomized controlled trials reported no difference between guanethidine and placebo.[9,15]

α-Adrenergic blockade with phentolamine also has been studied as a means to inhibit the sympathetic nervous system. It may be used as a placebo-controlled test to identify patients with SMP as a component of CRPS. It also has been used for treatment; however, in a double-blinded controlled study of patients with symptoms of SMP, phentolamine showed no efficacy compared to either placebo or an α-adrenergic agonist.[16,17]

Local anesthetic blockade of the sympathetic chain, known as stellate ganglion block when placed in the upper extremity, has become a standard in the diagnosis and treatment of CRPS type I. The use of these blocks is recommended for patients who are unable to participate in a functional rehabilitation program despite pharmacologic agents and have symptoms of SMP. Once prescribed, their efficacy should be carefully monitored. Both the effectiveness of the resultant sympathetic blockade and any improvement in pain should be documented to guide further treatment.

The sympathetic chain ganglions responsible for innervation of the hand and arm are found at the upper thoracic level, specifically at T2 and T3.[18] Blocks are typically given at C6 or C7 for safety and convenience, and the local anesthetic is expected to spread down to the thoracic ganglion. A Horner syndrome (characterized by ipsilateral ptosis, miosis, and anhidrosis) will occur with blockade anywhere along the cervical ganglion and does not necessarily indicate a successful upper thoracic block. Therefore, care must be taken to objectively measure signs of sympathetic block in the extremity (increase in skin temperature to at least 35°C), in addition to the presence of a Horner syndrome, to ensure an adequate sympathetic block is obtained.

Cepeda and associates[9] reviewed 29 studies regarding the efficacy of sympathetic blocks in the treatment of CRPS type I performed through 1999; only three of these were randomized controlled trials. The authors concluded that the support for efficacy of sympathetic blockade is based largely on retrospective case series that, by design, cannot control for the placebo effect. After pooling the outcome data, the average likelihood of achieving complete pain relief after sympathetic blockade was less than 33%, which is within the magnitude of the placebo response.[9]

Despite the lack of strong evidence supporting the use of sympathetic blockade, patient selection is critical. A block may help identify a sympathetically mediated component of the patient's pain and provide treatment. However, blocks should be continued only for patients who experience significant pain relief and only for as long as the benefit continues. In patients who report more than 50% improvement in symptom relief for at least 2 days following the block, a series of blocks is warranted. Some patients will have lasting pain relief following a series of blocks, and this relief is sufficient enough to allow others to regain function through physical therapy.

If sympathetic blockade fails to relieve pain and the patient reports inadequate pain control, neuromodulation techniques may be beneficial. The use of implantable peripheral nerve and spinal cord stimulators has become increasingly popular in recent years. One small, prospective randomized study reported that patients with CRPS who received spinal cord stimulation with physical therapy achieved greater pain relief and improvement in health-related quality-of-life measures compared with patients receiving physical therapy alone.[19]

Additional studies are necessary to identify effective treatments for CRPS type I. Until more evidence is available, a stepwise approach to treatment is advised, with the eventual goal of functional rehabilitation of the arm. Physical therapy should begin early, with the initial goals of edema control, gentle mobilization, and desensitization. Pharmacologic agents are added and adjusted as necessary. Patients should be reevaluated every 7 to 14 days to determine the effectiveness of pharmacologic treatment, and changes should be made as necessary to enable the patient to participate in the rehabilitation of the affected arm. Stellate ganglion blocks should be added early for patients with signs and symptoms of sympathetic overactivity. If the block is effective (ie, temperature in the limb higher than 35°C or 1.5°C more than the opposite limb, pres-

ence of a Horner syndrome, and pain relief), additional blocks are indicated. If the patient does not respond, the blocks should be discontinued. Finally, a multidisciplinary approach is often best, involving orthopaedist, physical therapist, pain management specialist, and psychotherapist.

CRPS Type II

Symptoms of CRPS associated with an identifiable nerve lesion are classified as CRPS type II (causalgia). Treatment is identical to that for CRPS type I, with the addition of treatment for the identifiable nerve lesion. Entrapped nerves should be released. If significant scar is present in the nerve bed, the addition of a fat flap, omental flap, or vein wrapping is beneficial. Neuromas are initially treated with aggressive desensitization. If significant localized pain continues, resection and implantation into muscle or bone is performed.

Acute Carpal Tunnel Syndrome

Although the carpal tunnel is open at both ends, it functions as a closed compartment. Following wrist trauma and fracture, the resulting hemorrhage and edema can induce an acute compartment syndrome within the carpal tunnel. With increasing pressures in the carpal tunnel, capillary blood flow to the median nerve is reduced and ultimately blocked, resulting in decrease or loss of median nerve motor and sensory function. The pressure above which nerve viability is threatened, known as the critical pressure threshold, has been identified as greater than 40 mm Hg in normotensive patients or within 30 mm Hg of the diastolic blood pressure.[20]

The time between fracture and onset of median nerve symptoms is important to document. The median nerve is at risk for contusion, traction injury, or laceration because of its proximity to the distal radius. If paresthesias develop immediately following fracture, direct injury should be suspected. However, if the patient reports the onset of paresthesias several hours after injury, or following a closed reduction, acute carpal tunnel syndrome should be suspected. In a prospective study, Dresing and associates[21] reported that carpal tunnel pressures in patients with distal radius fractures increased as a result of progressive fracture hematoma and attempts at reduction maneuvers. Specifically, initial pressure was 23 mm Hg, which increased to 44 mm Hg following reduction, then decreased to 37 mm Hg after 4 hours, and 26 mm Hg after 12 hours.

Wrist position also alters carpal tunnel pressures. In a study of 23 distal radius fractures, Gelberman and associates[22] measured pressures before reduction with the wrist in neutral, 20° of flexion, 40° of flexion, and 20° of extension. They recorded mean pressures of 18 mm Hg in neutral, 27 mm Hg with 20° of flexion, 47 mm Hg with 40° of flexion, and 35 mm Hg with 20° of extension. External compression is also known to elevate intracompartmental pressures. Circumferential casts and soft dressings can contribute to compartment syndromes. Finally, the placement of a hematoma block with local anesthetic has been shown to increase the pressure within the carpal tunnel.[23]

All patients with wrist trauma should be questioned about the presence of paresthesias and undergo careful sensibility testing. Two common and effective methods to assess sensibility are static two-point discrimination and Semmes-Weinstein monofilament testing. Semmes-Weinstein testing is more sensitive to gradual changes in nerve function, whereas static two-point discrimination may not be diminished unless nerve injury is more severe.[24]

In patients with distal radius fracture and progressive median nerve dysfunction, initial management should consist of gentle realignment of the limb into neutral wrist position, splinting, and elevation. The timing of surgical decompression is much debated.[24,25] Conservative recommendations specify observation for 24 to 48 hours, with decompression if symptoms persist. Others recommend decompression on diagnosis because poor outcomes have been reported with delayed decompression.[24,25] I prefer surgical decompression if the condition is present before any reduction maneuver. If paresthesias are present after a closed reduction, the splint and dressing are split down to the skin, the limb elevated, and careful serial examinations performed. If symptoms fail to improve or become worse over the next 6 to 12 hours, then I perform surgical decompression.

If the etiology of median nerve dysfunction (carpal tunnel syndrome versus contusion) is in doubt, pressure measurements should be obtained in the carpal tunnel for definitive diagnosis. If the absolute pressure is greater than 40 mm Hg or within 30 mm Hg of the diastolic pressure, carpal tunnel release should be performed.

Late Carpal Tunnel Syndrome

Carpal tunnel syndrome also can present as a late complication of distal radius fracture. It has been shown to be statistically related to fracture malunion. Collapse of the radius, with or without dorsal angulation, was a significant risk factor for late median nerve dysfunction.[26] Additional factors include volar callus, perineural scarring, and residual swelling. Depending on the severity of the malunion, correctional osteotomy may be necessary, in addition to transverse carpal ligament release, for complete decompression of the median nerve.

Direct Nerve Injury

Primary injury to the median, ulnar, and superficial radial nerves is uncommon. The median nerve is located 3 mm superficial to the distal aspect of the radius. It is susceptible to contusion, entrapment, and laceration, particularly with high-energy injuries. Lateral radiographs should be carefully reviewed for the presence of a volarly displaced fragment both before and after reduction. If the patient has persistent symptoms of median nerve dysfunction and a volarly displaced bone fragment, surgical carpal tunnel release with concomitant fracture reduction and fragment excision or repair, is indicated.

Ulnar neuropathy is less common after fractures of the distal radius. The ulnar nerve is found approximately 3 mm from the volar surface of the ulna at the wrist. It is particularly vulnerable with displaced ulnar neck and head fractures, with fractures involving the volar-ulnar corner of the distal radius, and in cases of distal radioulnar joint subluxation and/or dislocation. The ulnar nerve is thought to be protected from injury because of its increased excursion at the wrist in comparison with the median nerve.[27,28] Late ulnar nerve symptoms also may develop in association with soft-tissue scarring. Treatment of acute injury consists of gentle realignment of the fracture, splinting, and elevation. Patients with persistent symptoms or delayed diagnosis should be treated with decompression of the ulnar nerve through the ulnar tunnel and fracture site.

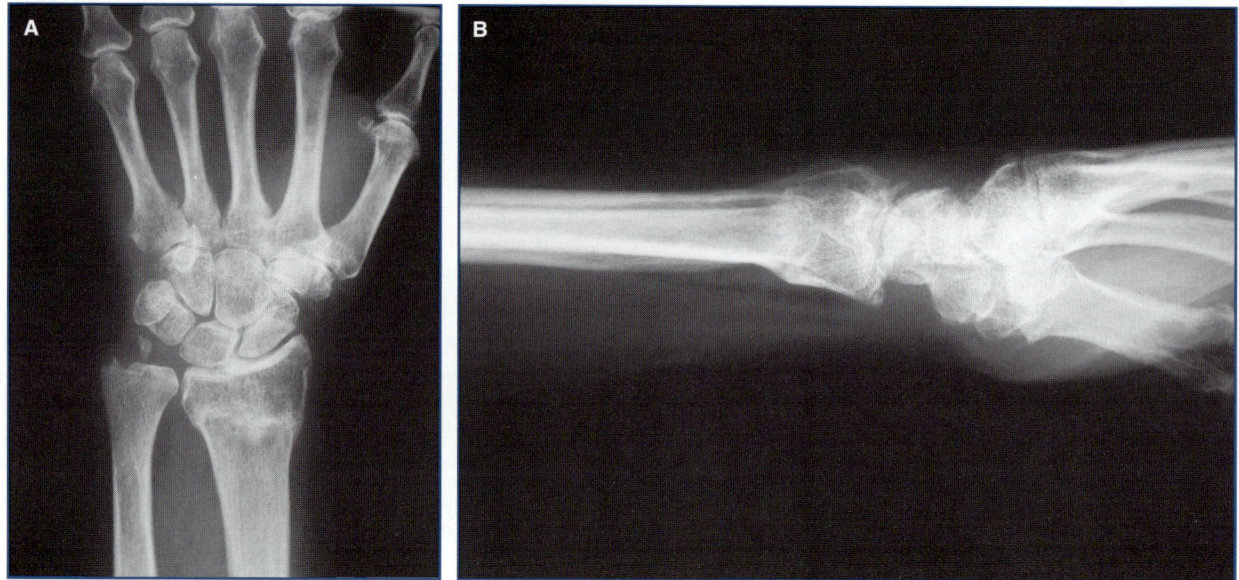

Figure 7 PA **(A)** and lateral **(B)** radiographs 6 months after surgery showing increased periarticular osteopenia.

Injuries to the branches of the superficial radial nerve are even more rare but occur principally as a result of external pressure from a cast or splint.[29,30] Therefore, bony prominences must be adequately padded, particularly the radial and ulnar styloids and the dorsum of the thumb. When identified, the offending splint or cast must be modified and aggressive desensitization of the area initiated. The other major cause of radial neuritis is a result of surgical treatment with K-wires or external fixation devices and is described elsewhere in this monograph.

MANAGEMENT AND OUTCOME SUMMARY

The patient presented for a second opinion 5.5 weeks after surgical repair of a distal radius fracture, with classic signs and symptoms of CRPS type I. She had no identifiable nerve injury or other reason for her symptoms. She was treated aggressively on the day she presented, with removal of her external fixator and K-wires, administration of a stellate ganglion block, and initiation of a physical therapy program. The stellate block was performed by an anesthesiologist. Skin temperature before the block was 33.7°C on the right side and 34.6°C on the left. After the stellate block,

skin temperature was 32.9°C on the right side and 37.3°C on the left. She noted decreased pain after a block of approximately 40%. A 1-week steroid taper was prescribed, and she continued to take narcotic medication on a scheduled basis.

Two additional stellate blocks were given within the next 4 days. She was seen in physical therapy 3 days a week and treated with aggressive edema control, stretching, taping of the digits, dynamic splinting, and a transcutaneous electrical nerve stimulator for pain relief (FDA device class 2). Over the next 3 months, the patient reported progressive improvements in pain, motion in her hand, and edema. She was weaned of narcotic analgesics after approximately 3 months. She recovered 80% of composite digital motion and functional wrist motion. Her distal radius fracture had healed with residual intra-articular incongruity, whereas the ulnar styloid fracture failed to unite (**Figure 7**). She continued to have limited shoulder motion with forward elevation of 130° and external rotation of 45°.

Her physical therapy program continued 2 to 3 days a week for several additional months. On final follow-up evaluation, 9 months after initial presentation, she reported occasional but tolerable pain. She had remained off pain medications and had regained near full shoulder motion.

REFERENCES

1. Stanton-Hicks M, Janig W, Hassenbusch S, et al: Reflex sympathetic dystrophy: Changing concepts and taxonomy. *Pain* 1995; 63:127-133.

2. Bruehl S, Harden RN, Galer BS, et al: External validation of IASP diagnostic criteria for Complex Regional Pain Syndrome and proposed research diagnostic criteria: International Association for the Study of Pain. *Pain* 1999;81:147-154.

3. Harden RN, Bruehl S, Galer BS, et al: Complex regional pain syndrome: Are the IASP diagnostic criteria valid and sufficiently comprehensive? *Pain* 1999;83:211-219.

4. Field J, Atkins RM: Algodystrophy is an early complication of Colles' fracture: What are the implications? *J Hand Surg [Br]* 1997;22: 178-182.

5. Atkins RM, Duckworth T, Kanis JA: Features of algodystrophy after Colles' fracture. *J Bone Joint Surg Br* 1990;72:105-110.

6. Veldman PH, Reynen HM, Arntz IE, Goris RJ: Signs and symptoms of reflex sympathetic dystrophy: Prospective study of 829 patients. *Lancet* 1993;342:1012-1016.

7. Bickerstaff DR, Kanis JA: Algodystrophy: An underrecognized complication of minor trauma. *Br J Rheumatol* 1994;33:240-248.

8. Zyluk A: The natural history of post-traumatic reflex sympathetic dystrophy. *J Hand Surg [Br]* 1998; 23:20-23.

9. Cepeda MS, Lau J, Carr DB: Defining the therapeutic role of local anesthetic sympathetic blockade in complex regional pain syndrome: A narrative and systematic review. *Clin J Pain* 2002;18:216-233.

10. Lee GW, Weeks PM: The role of bone scintigraphy in diagnosing reflex sympathetic dystrophy. *J Hand Surg [Am]* 1995;20:458-463.

11. Raja SN, Grabow TS: Complex regional pain syndrome I (reflex sympathetic dystrophy). *Anesthesiology* 2002;96:1254-1260.

12. Stanton-Hicks M, Baron R, Boas R, et al: Complex regional pain syndromes: Guidelines for therapy. *Clin J Pain* 1998;14:155-166.

13. Adami S, Fossaluzza V, Gatti D, Fracassi E, Braga V: Bisphosphonate therapy of reflex sympathetic dystrophy syndrome. *Ann Rheum Dis* 1997;56:201-204.

14. Kingery WS: A critical review of controlled clinical trials for peripheral neuropathic pain and complex regional pain syndromes. *Pain* 1997;73:123-139.

15. Livingstone JA, Atkins RM: Intravenous regional guanethidine blockade in the treatment of post-traumatic complex regional pain syndrome type 1 (algodystrophy) of the hand. *J Bone Joint Surg Br* 2002;84:380-386.

16. Verdugo RJ, Campero M, Ochoa JL: Phentolamine sympathetic block in painful polyneuropathies: II. Further questioning of the concept of 'sympathetically maintained pain'. *Neurology* 1994;44:1010-1014.

17. Verdugo RJ, Ochoa JL: Sympathetically maintained pain: I. Phentolamine block questions the concept. *Neurology* 1994;44:1003-1010.

18. Manning DC: Reflex sympathetic dystrophy, sympathetically maintained pain, and complex regional pain syndrome: Diagnoses of inclusion, exclusion, or confusion? *J Hand Ther* 2000;13:260-268.

19. Kemler MA, Barendse GA, van Kleef M, et al: Spinal cord stimulation in patients with chronic reflex sympathetic dystrophy. *New Engl J Med* 2000;343:618-624.

20. Gelberman RH, Szabo RM, Williamson RV, et al: Tissue pressure threshold for peripheral nerve viability. *Clin Orthop* 1983;178:285-291.

21. Dresing K, Peterson T, Schmit-Neuerburg KP: Compartment pressure in the carpal tunnel in distal fractures of the radius: A prospective study. *Arch Orthop Trauma Surg* 1994;113:285-289.

22. Gelberman RH, Szabo RM, Mortensen WW: Carpal tunnel pressures and wrist position in patients with Colles' fractures. *J Trauma* 1984;24:747-749.

23. Kongsholm J, Olerud C: Carpal tunnel pressure in the acute phase after Colles' fracture. *Arch Orthop Trauma Surg* 1986;105:183-186.

24. Szabo RM: Acute carpal tunnel syndrome. *Hand Clin* 1998;14: 419-429.

25. Ford DJ, Ali MS: Acute carpal tunnel syndrome: Complications of delayed decompression. *J Bone Joint Surg Br* 1986;68:758-759.

26. Aro H, Koivunen T, Katevuo K, Nieminen S, Aho AJ: Late compression neuropathies after Colles' fractures. *Clin Orthop* 1988;233: 217-225.

27. Vance RM, Gelberman RH: Acute ulnar neuropathy with fractures at the wrist. *J Bone Joint Surg Am* 1978;60:962-965.

28. Clarke AC, Spencer RF: Ulnar nerve palsy following fractures of the distal radius: Clinical and anatomical studies. *J Hand Surg [Br]* 1991;16:438-440.

29. Stewart HD, Innes AR, Burke FD: The hand complications of Colles' fractures. *J Hand Surg [Br]* 1985; 10:103-106.

30. Kozin SH, Wood MB: Early soft-tissue complications after distal radius fractures. *Instr Course Lect* 1993;42:89-98.

Chapter 6

Hardware Complications

Colby P. Young, MD

Case Presentation
Case 1

A 76-year-old retired woman sustained a low-energy fracture after a fall onto her outstretched left arm. She was referred to the office 1 week after closed reduction and cast immobilization. **Figure 1** demonstrates a poorly molded cast lacking an appropriate three-point molding technique of fracture stabilization in which the soft-tissue bridge is under tension. This contributed to the fracture collapse, significant dorsal angulation, and subluxation of the carpus, with the appearance of early midcarpal static instability.

Case 2

A right-handed 56-year-old woman who sustained a distal radius fracture was treated with closed reduction and radioulnar pinning at an outside facility. She was referred because of concern over early fracture collapse and loss of reduction. Her chief symptoms were pain and unacceptable cosmesis. Examination revealed obvious clinical deformity and loss of forearm motion, and her arm was fixed in slight pronation. In addition, she described paresthesias about the superficial radial nerve distribution distal to the pin sites. Loss of radial inclination is seen on the PA radiograph (**Figure 2**).

Discussion

Fractures involving the distal radius are described as the most common long bone fractures.[1] It is estimated that distal radius fractures account for 16% of all fractures[2] and one sixth of the fractures treated in emergency departments.[3] Early studies showed permanent loss of function in 24% of patients treated.[4] Despite the prevalence of this injury, complications and their management are rarely addressed. This lack may be, in part, a result of the numerous treatment options available, absence of specific fracture classifications for treatment,[5] and lack of standardized methods for treatment.[6]

Closed reduction and cast immobilization,[4] Kirschner wire (K-wire) fixation,[7] external fixation,[8] and open reduction and internal fixation (ORIF)[9] have been evaluated in various clinical settings as the primary treatment of distal

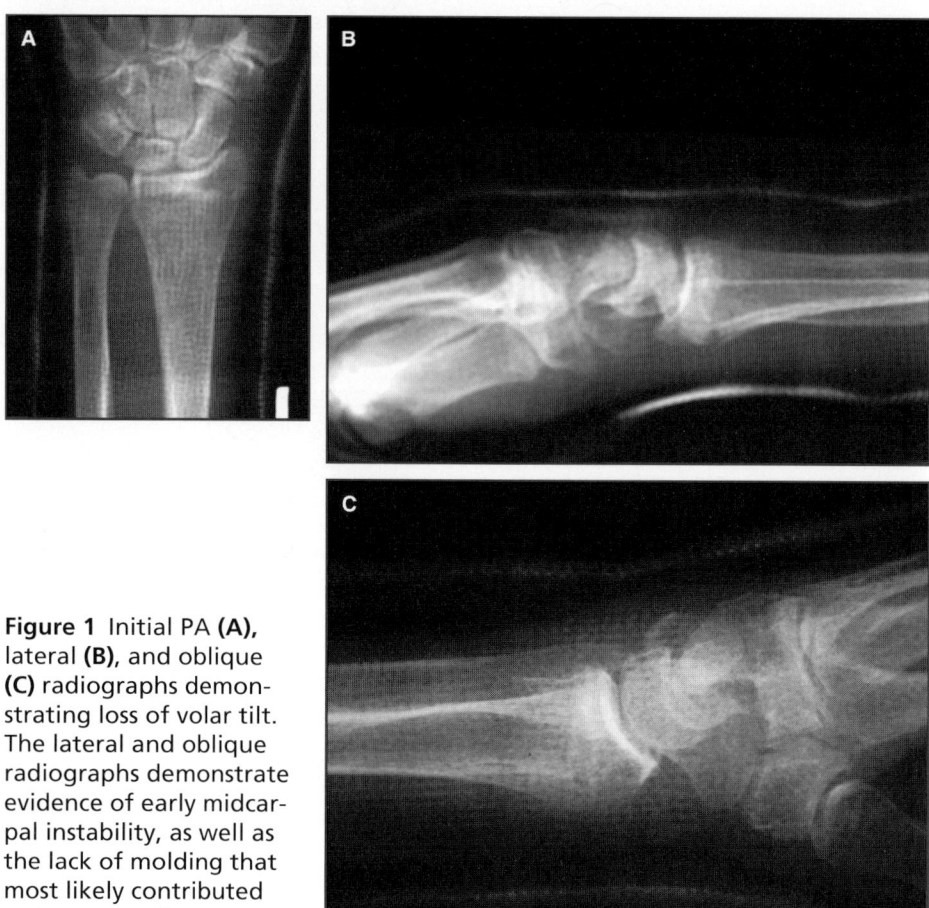

Figure 1 Initial PA **(A)**, lateral **(B)**, and oblique **(C)** radiographs demonstrating loss of volar tilt. The lateral and oblique radiographs demonstrate evidence of early midcarpal instability, as well as the lack of molding that most likely contributed to fracture collapse.

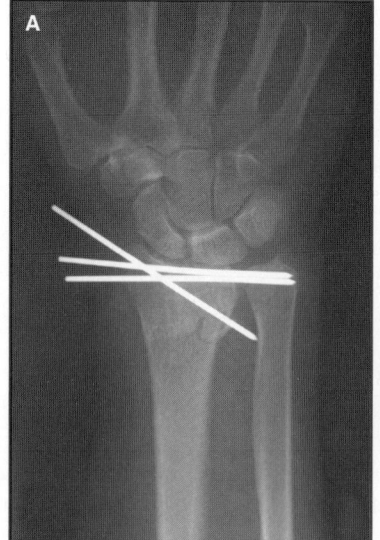

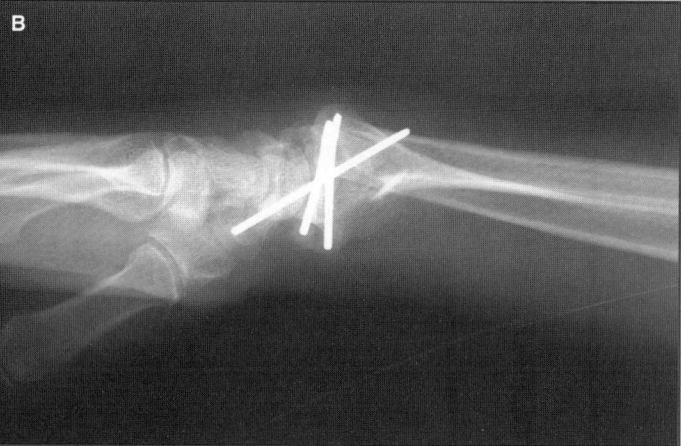

Figure 2 PA **(A)** and lateral **(B)** radiographs at presentation show loss of radial inclination on the PA radiograph.

radius fractures. The patient's functional and loading demands, work status, associated medical conditions, handedness, and cosmesis play a role in clinical decision making. In addition, bone quality, fracture stability, degree of comminution, and inherent bony stability are evaluated before selecting the appropriate course of action.[10] Goals of treatment are to maximize functional outcome and patient satisfaction while minimizing complications and poor results. As with any invasive technique, complications may occur.

Cast Immobilization

Closed reduction and cast immobilization has been advocated as the treatment of choice for most stable extra-articular fractures.[4,11] Loss of reduction is a common problem associated with cast immobilization. Although cast immobilization is successful in young patients with strong cortical and metaphyseal bone, collapse is more frequent in older, osteoporotic patients. Malunion has been reported in up to 60% of patients.[12] In a study evaluating redisplacement after closed reduction and splint immobilization, Abbaszadegan and associates[13] reported that loss of reduction frequently occurred between weeks 1 and 3. A total of 17% of the patients in this series were excluded because of a loss of reduction that required surgical treatment. The authors defined significant late displacement as loss of at least 3 mm of length or increased dorsal angulation of more than 10° after day 11. Of the remaining fractures, 7% met these criteria. In a separate study, these authors evaluated factors that predicted a poor result with re-reduction and found the amount of radial axial shortening and patient age were major prognostic factors.[14] After closed reduction and immobilization of fractures at risk, weekly follow-up for the first 3 postoperative weeks has been recommended to help identify and treat loss of reduction expeditiously. Although attempted re-reduction has been advocated, its benefits have been questioned, particularly in the elderly.[15,16] McQueen and associates[17] noted that after re-reduction in patients older than age 60 years, the mean dorsal angle improved on average less than 1°.

Other complications attributed to cast immobilization include soft-tissue necrosis, compartment syndrome, and neurovascular injury.[18,19] Skin necrosis and thermal burns may be avoided by placing adequate cast padding over areas of pressure. Skin surface pressure also has been evaluated in fiberglass and plaster casts. With the standard application technique (keeping the roll in contact with the limb), fiberglass-cast application was found to generate higher skin pressures than associated plaster-cast application. In addition, fiberglass was found to accommodate swelling poorly. By altering the application to a stretch-relax technique (pulling the roll of fiberglass away from the limb), tension was decreased and pressures were reduced, generating lower skin pressures than plaster casting.[20] By appropriate cast padding, delay of circumferential cast placement, and proper cast application technique,[21] these problems can be minimized. Judicious soft-tissue monitoring, weekly follow-up of fractures at risk, and the early conversion to more rigid fixation, if needed, also may help decrease complications.

Kirschner Wire Fixation

K-wire fixation has been an effective means of treating distal radius fractures since its initial description in 1908.[22] It has been advocated in the treatment of unstable, extra-articular, and minimally displaced intra-articular fractures of the distal radius.[10] The cortical bone should be primarily intact because the metaphyseal bone provides minimal stability.[23] Pin fixation has been shown to provide more stability, including both torsional rigidity and bending stiffness, than cast immobilization alone.[24]

Several variations in the technique, including percutaneous styloid pin fixation, intrafocal and extrafocal pin fixation, and ulnar-radial pinning, have been previously described.[22] Complications associated with K-wire fixation include cutaneous nerve and vessel injury, attritional rupture of tendons, chronic regional pain syndrome (CRPS), pin migration, pin fracture, irritation, and loss of reduction.[25-28] An anecdotal case report describes pin migration to the heart.[29]

K-wire fixation, in its various forms, is frequently performed percutaneously. The percutaneous technique was compared with the limited open technique in two separate cadaveric studies.[30,31] Steinberg and associates[31] demonstrated a safe zone of pin fixation (**Figure 3**), and Hochwald and associates[30] demonstrated the close proximity of cutaneous nerves and vessels and frequent injury to these structures. Both advocate a limited open technique for minimizing the risk of injury. Limited open techniques also allow for

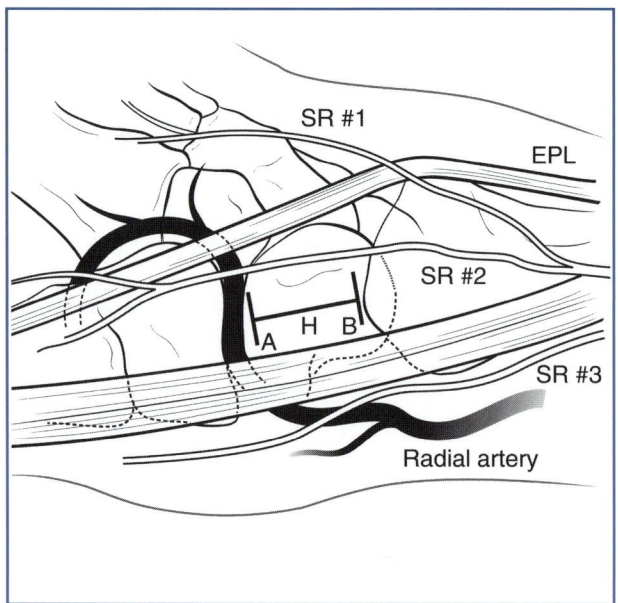

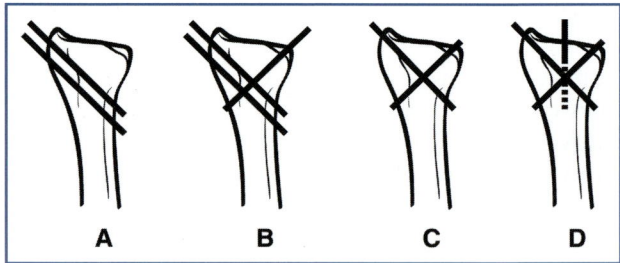

Figure 4 Pin configurations tested. Configuration A had two styloid pins; B had two styloid pins and one ulnar corner pin; C had two cross-pins; and D had two cross pins and one dorsovolar pin. Configuration B was the most stable construct. (Adapted with permission from Naidu SH, Bixler B, Capo JT, Moulton MJ, Radin A: Percutaneous pinning of distal radius fractures: A biomechanical study. *J Hand Surg [Am]* 1997; 22:252-257.)

Figure 3 The formula for a trapezoid, 1/2 (A+B) × H, was used to calculate the safe zone bounded by the radial artery, the SR2 branch (superficial radial nerve branch 2), the first dorsal compartment, and the radial styloid, where H is the distance from the radial styloid to the radial artery, A is the distance of the extensor pollicis brevis (EPB) to the SR 2 branch at the radial artery; and B is the distance from the EPB to the SR2 branch at the radial styloid. EPL = extensor pollicis longus. (Adapted with permission from Steinberg BD, Plancher KD, Idler RS: Percutaneous Kirschner wire fixation through the snuff box: An anatomic study. *J Hand Surg [Am]* 1995;20:57-62.)

evaluation of pin proximity to tendons so that attritional irritation can be minimized.

Another frequent complication involving pin fixation is loss of reduction.[32] Loss of reduction has been reported as high as 26%.[27] Naidu and associates[24] evaluated both pin configuration and pin number in unstable extra-articular bending fractures. In an in vitro biomechanical study evaluating the size (0.045 to 0.078 in) and configuration of pins (**Figure 4**), the authors reported that after evaluating six different constructs, two radial styloid pins and one ulnar corner pin provided the most rigid construct. Pin size of 0.062 in was found to adequately stabilize the fractures. Larger pins (0.078 in) demonstrated increased torsional stability but provided no increase in bending

stability.[31] Average time for pin removal ranged from 6 to 8 weeks; however, Rayhack[22] cautions that union may not be present in patients with dorsal comminution or osteoporosis, even at 8 weeks. Complications with this technique are reported to be less frequent than with more invasive techniques.[33]

External Fixation

Since its initial description by Anderson and O'Neil[34] in 1944, external fixation has been recognized as a treatment option for unstable extra-articular fractures, as well as for restoration of complex intra-articular distal radius fractures.[8,35-39] Its function is to maintain distraction and neutralize compressive loads by minimizing the displacing musculotendinous forces that allow collapse and shortening.[23] Radial length and inclination are believed to be restored via ligamentotaxis.[40] External fixation has little effect on reduction of volar tilt. The thick, strong V-shaped volar ligaments have been shown to reach maximum tension before the thinner Z-shaped dorsal ligaments. With longitudinal traction, this anatomic configuration predisposes a fracture to maintain dorsal tilt.[41] Bartosh and Saldana[41] further demonstrated that volar tilt was restored only after transection of the palmar ligaments. Even with its inability to control volar tilt, satisfactory results of up to 86% following external fixator application have been reported.

TABLE 1 Checketts and Otterburn Classification of Pin Tract Infection

Grade	Clinical Findings	Treatment
I	Slight discharge and redness around pin sites	Local wound care
II	Erythema involving the surrounding skin Involved skin is tender to palpation Purulence may or may not be present	Local wound care and oral antibiotics
III	Same as grade II except no improvement with local treatment and antibiotics	Requires pin removal and repositioning of affected pin at different location for resolution
IV	Severe soft tissue involvement at more than one pin site No improvement with local treatment	Pin removal and abandonment of external fixation
V	Same as grade IV except radiographic evidence of osteomyelitis	Same as grade IV
VI	Sequestrum present with persistent sinus	Abandonment of external fixation plus additional surgery required

Adapted with permission from Checketts RG, Otterburn M: Pin tract infection: Definition, prevention, incidence, in *Current Perspectives in External and Intramedullary Fixation: Abstracts of the 2nd Riva Congress.* Riva de Garda, Italy, University of Verona and University of Montpellier, 1992, pp 98-99.

Despite satisfactory treatment results, complications of up to 62% have been reported.[42] Complications associated with external fixation include pin tract infection, osteomyelitis, hardware loosening with subsequent loss of reduction, fracture, nerve injury, wrist and finger stiffness, and algodystrophy.[33,43,44]

Pin Site Complications

Pin insertion technique, pin design, bone quality, and demands on the pin are relevant to external fixation placement. Most pin problems associated with external fixation arise from the quality of the pin-bone interface.[45] Pin loosening and infection have been reported as the most common complication of external fixation, with studies demonstrating rates of up to 23%.[43,46] A frequent concern regarding loosening and infection is the need for predrilling half-size pins prior to their placement. In a recent study by Hutchinson and associates,[47] failure to predrill half pins resulted in higher bone thermal temperatures but not higher risk of complications. Judicious pin care, including daily cleansing of the pin sites, may help diminish the risk of pin tract infection. If pin tract infection develops, the early initiation of oral antibiotics is reported to help diminish sequelae associated with its use.[42] Checketts and Otterburn[48] developed a classification system regarding treatment of pin tract infection (**Table 1**).

The use of 3-mm diameter pins has been recommended for both the radius and the metacarpal. In evaluating adequate half-pin size, pins of 3-mm diameter demonstrated no fractures compared to 6% when pins of 2-mm diameter were used.[43] Moroni and associates[49] evaluated the use of hydroxyapatite-coated pins in patients with osteoporosis. Increased pullout strength and absence of gross loosening and pin tract infections were observed in osteoporotic patients treated with these pins. The use of three half pins per bone also has been advocated in patients with severe osteoporosis.[45]

Overdistraction

Acceptable distraction is a point of contention among authors. Despite conflicting reports regarding its merit, overdistraction has been associated with wrist and finger stiffness, CRPS, and nonunion.[33,50,51] Intraoperative ability to passively allow full composite digital flexion has been recommended as a clinical indicator of acceptable distraction. Biyani[52] evaluated 7 of 32 patients treated with external fixation who had more than 5 mm of distraction. He found that the amount of distraction did not significantly alter the final outcome. Maintenance of a normal distal radioulnar relationship was more important than distraction in final outcome. Excessive tension was evaluated in a cadaver model by Gupta and associates.[46] In distracting the wrist of cadavers from 0 to 50 lb, full digital flexion was possible at all levels of tension. There was extrinsic tightness of the index finger at 20 lb of tension. The authors caution the use of composite digital flexion as an indicator of acceptable distraction.

Kaempffe and associates,[33] using the carpal height index,[53] objectively evaluated distraction. They found that pain, function, wrist motion, and grip strength were adversely affected proportionately to increasing carpal height index. Functional outcome was also found to be worse as duration of distraction increased. Their study did not quantify the point of maximum distraction leading to a poor result. Although increased tension improves reduction and radiographic appearance, the potential adverse effects outweigh the benefits.[33] Composite finger flexion should not be the only factor in acceptable distraction. Others have recommended limiting distraction to 1 to 2 mm to prevent nerve injury, CRPS, and finger stiffness.[54-56]

Pin Site Fracture

Fractures occurring at the site of pin insertion may be either iatrogenic or posttraumatic. Weber and Szabo[42] effectively treated this complication with closed reduction and cast immobilization for metacarpal fractures and ORIF of forearm fractures.

Loss of Reduction

Because external fixators are unable to adequately control volar tilt, several alternatives have been described. Agee[57] recognized that palmar translation was required to restore and maintain volar tilt. He advocated use of a multiplanar external fixator to restore volar tilt. Its ability to control sagittal plane translation has been seen as a benefit.

The use of supplemental K-wires also has been proved to provide increased support and to assist with restoration of volar tilt. Several studies have demonstrated the benefit of augmenting an external fixator with supplemental K-wires.[55,58-61] In addition, external fixation accompanied by bone graft (either autograft or allograft) has been beneficial in preventing loss of reduction.[2,62-64]

Cosmesis

Patient dissatisfaction with external fixator cosmesis also has been reported.[43] Patient complaints include pin site keloid and painful scar formation. This problem may be of particular concern in those who develop hypertrophic scar. Patients should be cautioned of this potential prior to implementation.

Open Reduction and Internal Fixation

The importance of a congruent articular surfaces to prevent or delay posttraumatic osteoarthritis is described in the literature.[9,65-69] Several series advocate articular restoration when step-off is greater than 1 to 2 mm in an attempt to decrease the risk of posttraumatic osteoarthritis.[70-72] Potential indications for ORIF include displaced intra-articular fractures,[9,67,73] marginal shear fractures,[74-76] and unstable, bending fractures that have failed nonsurgical management.[77,78] Internal fixation has the advantage of restoring articular congruity of small fracture fragments, potentially allowing early range-of-motion (ROM) exercises. Early ROM exercises improve healing of articular cartilage[79] and limit potential capsular and ligamentous adhesions that may indicate a less than satisfactory result.[80] Dorsal plate fixation and, more recently, volar plate systems have been advocated to achieve this goal.

Dorsal Plate Fixation

Traditional methods of internal fixation rely on dorsal plating systems to restore articular congruity, radial height, inclination, and volar tilt.[9] Early plate design has led to difficulty with fashioning and contouring the plate.[81,82] In this situation, the intervening hardware is in close proximity to adjacent tendons because of the paucity of intervening soft tissue between the bone and the extensor mechanism (**Figure 5**). Adequate repair of the extensor retinaculum for plate coverage is often difficult, potentiating the risk of tendon irritation and subsequent rupture. In addition, prominent screw heads have led to further soft-tissue complications.[83]

Despite acceptable results in several series,[9,66,72,81,84] dorsal plate fixation has been associated with compli-

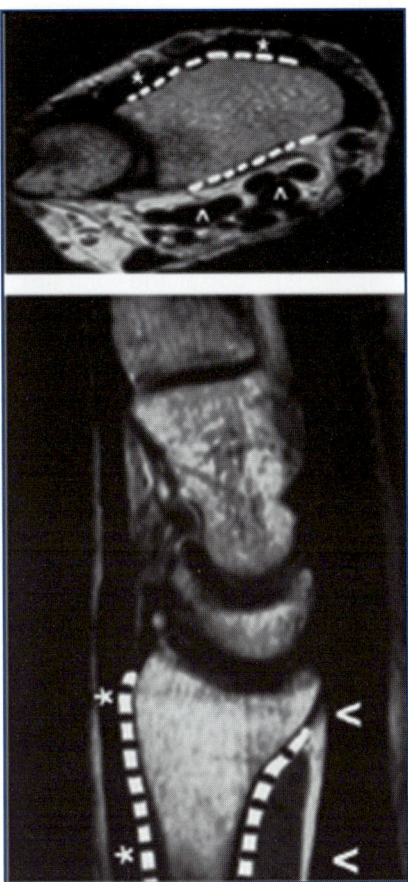

Figure 5 Interrupted lines represent plate application sites on these MRI images. **A,** Dorsal tendons (*) directly contact the dorsal plate. **B,** Volar tendons (arrowheads) are well separated from the volar plate by the pronator quadratus. (Adapted with permission from Orbay JL, Fernandez DL: Volar fixation for dorsally displaced fractures of the distal radius: A preliminary report. *J Hand Surg [Am]* 2002;27:205-215.)

cation rates up to 63%.[65,72,85] Extensor tenosynovitis and tendon rupture,[84,86] loss of reduction,[77] and painful hardware requiring removal have been shown to be potential complications.[87]

Tendon irritation and rupture are reported as the most common complications associated with dorsal plating.[86] In a small retrospective study evaluating complications of the Pi plate (Synthes, West Chester, PA) in distal radius fractures and corrective osteotomies, 63% of patients were found to have tendon irritation. Plate removal was recommended if patients

had dorsal wrist pain.[88] In a recent study evaluating dorsal plating, the Pi plate was compared to various low-profile plates. Hardware removal or tendon reconstruction was required in 47% of patients treated with the Pi plate. None of the low-profile plates required removal. There was no difference in complications related to the biomaterial composition of the plate (stainless steel versus titanium). All complications were associated with tendon irritation and attritional rupture. Despite the high complication rate, the outcome was cited as good or excellent in all patients according to the Gartland and Werley scoring system.[86] Tenosynovitis and plate irritation prior to rupture have been treated with corticosteroid injection, splint immobilization, retinacular flap coverage of the hardware, or plate removal alone or in combination. Retinacular flap coverage failed to prevent dorsal wrist pain in 45% of patients, and Chiang and associates[88] recommend routine plate removal when dorsal wrist pain is present to prevent tendon ruptures.

Tendon rupture, including both flexor and extensor tendon systems, has been seen as a result of excessively long screws and inappropriately placed plates.[87,89-91] Tendon rupture has been adequately treated with interpositional tendon grafting or tendon transfers.[85,86,88] If the treating surgeon is unfamiliar with these techniques, hand surgery referral is prudent at this juncture of treatment.

Volar Plating of Dorsally Displaced Distal Radius Fractures

Because of the complications associated with dorsal plating, an innovative approach to dorsally displaced fractures using a volar fixed-angle plate has been described.[78,92] Benefits of this technique include a large protective soft-tissue envelope (**Figure 5**) and less risk of tenosynovitis and tendon rupture.[93]

Orbay,[78] in a preliminary report of 31 patients evaluated at a minimum of 1 year, found only one patient to have extensor tenosynovitis resulting from a long support peg. This problem was treated with hardware removal. No other complications were reported. Jupiter and associates[77] and Keating and associates[94] both reported that dorsal displacement may occur as a result of inadequate integrity of the dorsal metaphyseal cortex when volar plate fixation is used. The loss of adequate metaphyseal bone stock contrib-

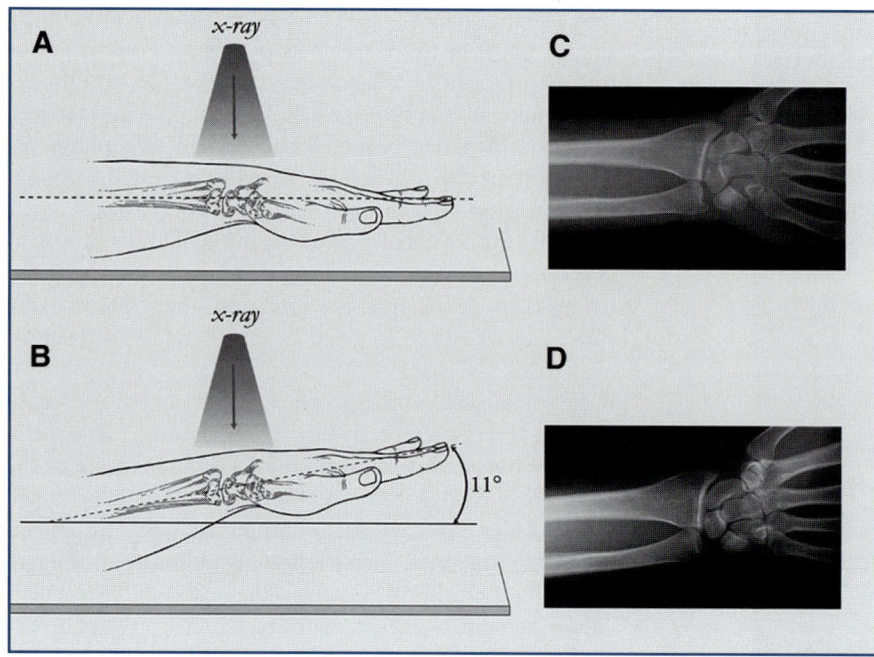

Figure 6 A, Standard PA wrist position and radiograph. The dorsal lip of the distal radius (arrowheads) is superimposed on the proximal aspect of the lunate and scaphoid. **B,** Anatomic tilt (11°) PA wrist position and radiograph. The radiograph is tangential to the dorsal and volar lips of the distal radius. **C,** Radiograph produced by standard PA positioning. **D,** Radiograph produced by anatomic tilt position. The dorsal and volar lips of the radius more nearly overlap each other. (Adapted with permission from Boyer MI, Korcek KJ, Gelberman RH, et al: Anatomic tilt x-rays of the distal radius: An ex vivo analysis of surgical fixation. *J Hand Surg [Am]* 2004;29:116-122.)

utes to this position because load is borne across the radiocarpal joint. Orbay and Fernandez[95] describe placing the fixed-angle support pegs in the most distal subchondral bone possible to help prevent settling. They found only 1 to 2 mm loss of radial length when using this technique in patients with osteoporosis. The position was deemed acceptable provided the capitate, lunate, and radius alignment was acceptable.[77]

When placing subchondral screws or pegs close to the articular surface in the subchondral bone, normal PA and lateral radiographs may give the inaccurate appearance of intra-articular screw extension. An 11° volar tilt and a 23° lateral radiograph have been shown to be superior to normal PA and lateral radiographs in evaluating appropriate subchondral screw placement[96] (**Figures 6** and **7**).

Arthroscopic-Assisted Treatment of Distal Radius Fractures

Continued advancements in the treatment of intra-articular distal radius fractures have led to arthroscopic joint surface evaluation. Arthroscopy has a number of benefits over formal arthrotomy. Arthroscopy provides direct visualization of the biconcave

articular surface, potentially obviating the need for arthrotomy. Associated soft-tissue injuries may be evaluated, osteochondral flaps and loose bodies may be removed, and capsular adhesions with resultant functional stiffness[97] may be avoided. In an evaluation of 60 patients with intra-articular distal radius fractures, 68% were found to have previously undetected soft-tissue injuries. These were found most frequently accompanying injuries to the lunate facet.[98]

Complications of this technique have been relatively minor and include transient neuritis. No cases of CRPS have been reported in several series. Contraindications include compartment syndrome, open joint injury, skin and soft-tissue contamination, and significant soft-tissue injury.

Bone Grafting

Corticocancellous autograft is traditionally used for filling metaphyseal voids and helping to restore radial height, length, and volar tilt. Iliac crest autograft has osteoinductive, osteoconductive, and osteogenic properties, but its harvest is associated with increased morbidity. Complications, including hematoma, fracture, infection, and neuritis, have been reported in up to

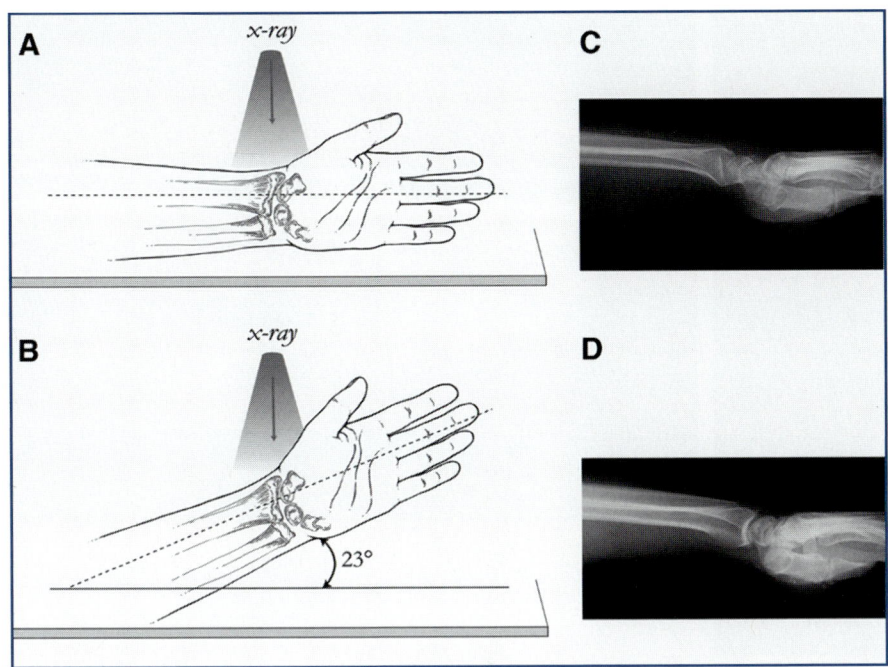

Figure 7 A, Standard lateral wrist position. **B,** Anatomic tilt (23°) lateral wrist position. The radiograph is exposed tangential to the distal radius articular surface. **C,** Radiograph produced by standard lateral position. The radial styloid is superimposed on the scaphoid. **D,** Radiograph produced by anatomic tilt position. Note subjective improvement in visualization of the subchondral bone of the distal radius articular surface. (Adapted with permission from Boyer MI, Korcek KJ, Gelberman RH, et al: Anatomic tilt x-rays of the distal radius: An ex vivo analysis of surgical fixation. *J Hand Surg [Am]* 2004;29:116-122.)

10% of patients.[99] The use of polymethylmethacrylate also has been reported with acceptable results.[100] However, concerns about intra-articular extravasation and the lack of osseous integration with the use of polymethylmethacrylate[101] have led to the consideration of bone graft substitutes.

Bone graft substitutes, either isolated or in conjunction with other means of fixation, have been shown to improve early clinical outcome. In a study comparing an injectable calcium phosphate versus external fixation, early functional results demonstrated a benefit to the use of calcium phosphate. At 1-year follow-up, clinical outcomes for grip strength and mobility were comparable.[102] Complications include extravasation of material into the articular surface, acute synovitis, and loss of reduction. In a study by Sanchez-Sotelo and associates,[101] the use of remodelable bone cement resulted in soft-tissue extrusion in initial evaluation 69% of the time. Although this extrusion most commonly resorbed, 32% of patients were found to have persistent extrusion at 1 year. Another concern regarding these products is the prolonged radiographic opacity. However, the long-term risks are unknown.[103]

MANAGEMENT AND OUTCOME SUMMARY
Case 1

The patient underwent closed reduction and limited open pin fixation. Informed consent was obtained. Intraoperative passive tenodesis was performed to ensure there was no binding of the extensor tendons. Cast immobilization was used to supplement pin fixation. Early digital ROM was begun, and the pins were removed at 8 weeks (**Figure 8**). Follow-up was uneventful with restoration of functional ROM, allowing full activities of daily living.

Case 2

Informed consent was obtained. The pins were subsequently removed, and plate fixation was performed. Early ROM was initiated. At the 10-week follow-up examination, the paresthesias had resolved, functional ROM was restored, and the patient had pain-free motion (**Figure 9**).

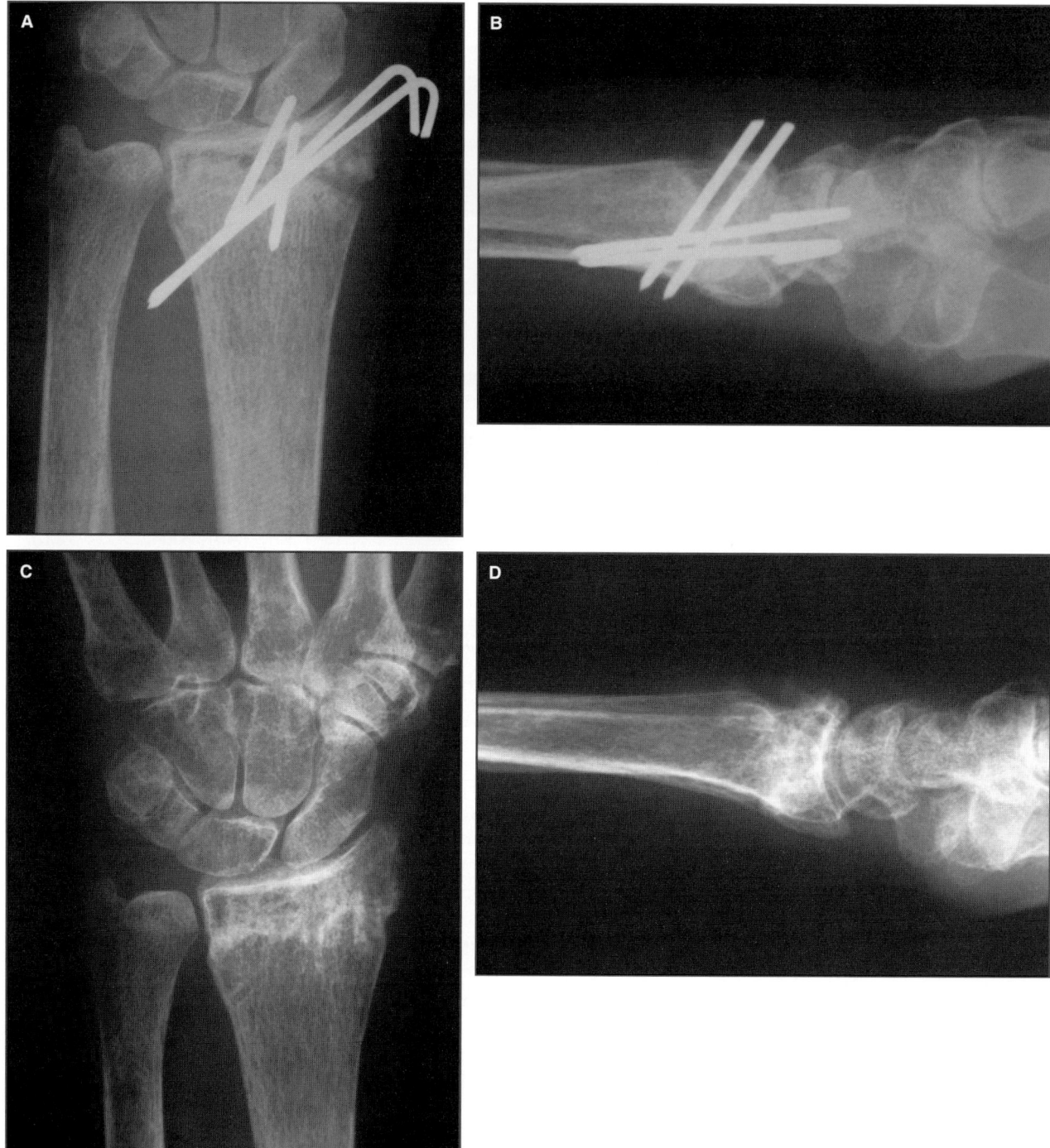

Figure 8 PA **(A)** and lateral **(B)** views after reduction. Note restoration of height, inclination, and neutral tilt. **C** and **D**, Maintenance of acceptable alignment at 3-month follow-up.

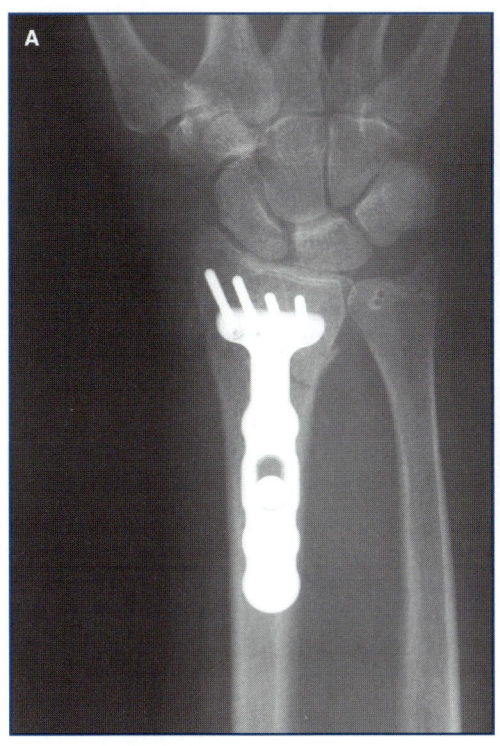

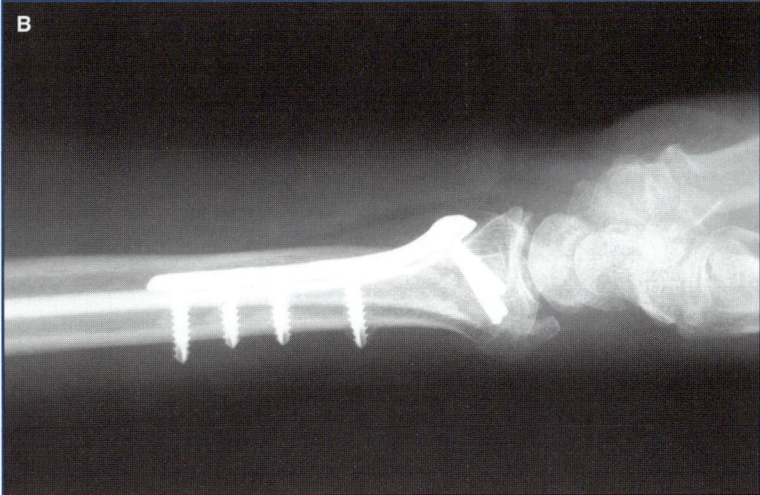

Figure 9 PA **(A)** and lateral **(B)** radiographs after ORIF. There is restoration of radial inclination, height, and tilt. Also note the position of the distal support pegs located in the subchondral bone.

REFERENCES

1. Werber KD, Raeder F, Brauer RB, Weiss S: External fixation of distal radial fractures: Four compared with five pins. A randomized prospective study. *J Bone Joint Surg Am* 2003;85:660-666.

2. Herrera M, Chapman CB, Rob M, Strauch RJ, Rosenwasser MP: Treatment of unstable distal radius fractures with cancellous allograft and external fixation. *J Hand Surg [Am]* 1999;24:1269-1278.

3. Ark J, Jupiter JB: The rationale for precise management of distal radius fractures. *Orthop Clin North Am* 1993;24:205-210.

4. Bacorn RW, Kurtzke JF: Colles' fracture: A study of two thousand cases from the New York State Workmen's Compensation Board. *J Bone Joint Surg Am* 1953;35:643-658.

5. Porter M, Stockley I: Fractures of the distal radius: Intermediate and end results in relation to radiologic parameters. *Clin Orthop* 1987;220:241-252.

6. Cooney WP III, Dobyns JH, Linscheid RL: Complications of Colles' fractures. *J Bone Joint Surg Am* 1980;62:613-619.

7. DePalma AF: Comminuted fractures of the distal end of the radius treated by ulnar pinning. *J Bone Joint Surg Am* 1952;34:651-662.

8. Cooney WP III, Linscheid RL, Dobyns JH: External pin fixation for unstable Colles' fractures. *J Bone Joint Surg Am* 1979;61:840-845.

9. Bradway JK, Amadio PC, Cooney WP: Open reduction and internal fixation of displaced, comminuted intra-articular fractures of the distal end of the radius. *J Bone Joint Surg Am* 1989;71:839-847.

10. Fernandez D, Jupiter JB: *Fractures of the Distal Radius: A Practical Approach to Management.* New York, NY, Springer-Verlag, 1996, pp 104-158.

11. Wahlstrom O: Treatment of Colles' fracture: A prospective comparison of three different positions of immobilization. *Acta Orthop Scand* 1982;53:225-228.

12. Gartland JJ Jr, Werley CW: Evaluation of healed Colles' fractures. *J Bone Joint Surg Am* 1951;33:895-907.

13. Abbaszadegan H, von Sivers K, Jonsson U: Late displacement of Colles' fractures. *Int Orthop* 1988;12:197-199.

14. Abbaszadegan H, Jonsson U, von Sivers K: Prediction of instability of Colles' fractures. *Acta Orthop Scand* 1989;60:646-650.

15. McQueen MM, Hajducka C, Court-Brown CM: Redisplaced

unstable fractures of the distal radius: A prospective randomised comparison of four methods of treatment. *J Bone Joint Surg Br* 1996;78:404-409.

16. Schmalholz A: Closed rereduction of axial compression in Colles' fracture is hardly possible. *Acta Orthop Scand* 1989;60:57-59.

17. McQueen MM, MacLaren A, Chalmers J: The value of remanipulating Colles' fractures. *J Bone Joint Surg Br* 1986;68: 232-233.

18. Field J, Atkins RM: Algodystrophy is an early complication of Colles' fracture: What are the implications? *J Hand Surg [Br]* 1997;22:178-182.

19. Field J, Protheroe DL, Atkins RM: Algodystrophy after Colles' fractures is associated with secondary tightness of casts. *J Bone Joint Surg Br* 1994;76:901-905.

20. Davids JR, Frick SL, Skewes E, Blackhurst DW: Skin surface pressure beneath an above-the-knee cast: Plaster casts compared with fiberglass casts. *J Bone Joint Surg Am* 1997;79:565-569.

21. Kozin SH, Wood MB: Early soft-tissue complications after fractures of the distal part of the radius. *J Bone Joint Surg Am* 1993;75:144-153.

22. Rayhack JM: The history and evolution of percutaneous pinning of displaced distal radius fractures. *Orthop Clin North Am* 1993;24:287-300.

23. Simic PM, Weiland AJ: Fractures of the distal aspect of the radius: Changes in treatment over the past two decades. *Instr Course Lect* 2003;52:185-195.

24. Naidu SH, Bixler B, Capo JT, Moulton MJ, Radin A: Percutaneous pinning of distal radius fractures: A biomechanical study. *J Hand Surg [Am]* 1997;22: 252-257.

25. Collicut J, Gross M, Johnson J: A biomechanical analysis of percu-taneous pinning for unstable extra-articular fractures of the distal radius. *J Bone Joint Surg Br* 1992;76(suppl 1):23.

26. Dowdy PA, Patterson SD, King GJ, Roth JH, Chess D: Intrafocal (Kapandji) pinning of unstable distal radius fractures: A preliminary report. *J Trauma* 1996;40: 194-198.

27. Greatting MD, Bishop AT: Intrafocal (Kapandji) pinning of unstable fractures of the distal radius. *Orthop Clin North Am* 1993;24:301-307.

28. Munson GO, Gainor BJ: Percutaneous pinning of distal radius fractures. *J Trauma* 1981;21: 1032-1035.

29. Seipel RC, Schmeling GJ, Daley RA: Migration of a K-wire from the distal radius to the heart. *Am J Orthop* 2001;30:147-151.

30. Hochwald NL, Levine R, Tornetta P III: The risks of Kirschner wire placement in the distal radius: A comparison of techniques. *J Hand Surg [Am]* 1997; 22:580-584.

31. Steinberg BD, Plancher KD, Idler RS: Percutaneous Kirschner wire fixation through the snuff box: An anatomic study. *J Hand Surg [Am]* 1995;20:57-62.

32. Mah ET, Atkinson RN: Percutaneous Kirschner wire stabilisation following closed reduction of Colles' fractures. *J Hand Surg [Br]* 1992;17:55-62.

33. Kaempffe FA, Wheeler DR, Peimer CA, et al: Severe fractures of the distal radius: Effect of amount and duration of external fixator distraction on outcome. *J Hand Surg [Am]* 1993;18: 33-41.

34. Anderson R, O'Neil G: Comminuted fractures of the distal end of the radius. *Surg Gynecol Obstet* 1944;78:434-440.

35. Kongsholm J, Olerud C: Plaster cast versus external fixation for unstable intraarticular Colles'

fractures. *Clin Orthop* 1989;241: 57-65.

36. Cooney WP: External fixation of distal radial fractures. *Clin Orthop* 1983;180:44-49.

37. Frykman GK, Tooma GS, Boyko K, Henderon R: Comparison of eleven external fixators for treatment of unstable wrist fractures. *J Hand Surg [Am]* 1989;14(2 Pt 1):247-254.

38. Nakata RY, Chaud Y, Matiko JD, Frykman GK, Wood VE: External fixators for wrist fractures: A biomechanical and clinical study. *J Hand Surg [Am]* 1985;10(6 Pt 1):845-851.

39. Vaughan PA, Lui SM, Harrington IJ, Maistrelli GL: Treatment of unstable fractures of the distal radius by external fixation. *J Bone Joint Surg Br* 1985;67: 385-389.

40. Melone CP Jr: Distal radius fractures: Patterns of articular fragmentation. *Orthop Clin North Am* 1993;24:239-253.

41. Bartosh RA, Saldana MJ: Intraarticular fractures of the distal radius: A cadaveric study to determine if ligamentotaxis restores radiopalmar tilt. *J Hand Surg [Am]* 1990;15:18-21.

42. Weber SC, Szabo RM: Severely comminuted distal radial fracture as an unsolved problem: Complications associated with external fixation and pins and plaster techniques. *J Hand Surg [Am]* 1986; 11:157-165.

43. Sanders RA, Keppel FL, Waldrop LI: External fixation of distal radial fractures: Results and complications. *J Hand Surg [Am]* 1991;16:385-391.

44. Green SA, Ripley MJ: Chronic osteomyelitis in pin tracks. *J Bone Joint Surg Am* 1984;66:1092-1098.

45. Schuind FA, Burny F, Chao EY: Biomechanical properties and design considerations in upper extremity external fixation. *Hand Clin* 1993;9:543-553.

46. Gupta R, Bozentka DJ, Bora FW: The evaluation of tension in an experimental model of external fixation of distal radius fractures. *J Hand Surg [Am]*1999;24: 108-112.

47. Hutchinson DT, Bachus KN, Higgenbotham T: External fixation of the distal radius: To predrill or not to predrill. *J Hand Surg [Am]* 2000;25:1064-1068.

48. Checketts RG, Otterburn M: Pin tract infection: Definition, prevention, incidence, in *Current Perspectives in External and Intramedullary Fixation: Abstracts of the 2nd Riva Congress.* Riva de Garda, Italy, University of Verona and University of Montpellier, 1992, pp 98-99.

49. Moroni A, Faldini C, Marchetti S, et al: Improvement of the bone-pin interface strength in osteoporotic bone with use of hydroxyapatite-coated tapered external-fixation pins: A prospective, randomized clinical study of wrist fractures. *J Bone Joint Surg Am* 2001;83:717-721.

50. Suso S, Combalia A, Segur JM, Garcia-Ramiro S, Roman R: Comminuted intra-articular fractures of the distal end of the radius treated with the Hoffmann external fixator. *J Trauma* 1993; 35:61-66.

51. Combalia A, Suso S: Reflex sympathetic dystrophy in severe fractures of the distal radius treated with distraction devices. *J Hand Surg [Am]* 1994;19:156-157.

52. Biyani A: Over-distraction of the radio-carpal and mid-carpal joints following external fixation of comminuted distal radial fractures. *J Hand Surg [Br]* 1993;18: 506-510.

53. Youm Y, McMurthy RY, Flatt AE, Gillespie TE: Kinematics of the wrist: I. An experimental study of radial-ulnar deviation and flexion-extension. *J Bone Joint Surg Am* 1978;60:423-431.

54. Seitz WH Jr: External fixation of distal radius fractures: Indications and technical principles. *Orthop Clin North Am* 1993;24:255-264.

55. Seitz WH Jr, Froimson AI, Leb R, Shapiro JD: Augmented external fixation of unstable distal radius fractures. *J Hand Surg [Am]* 1991;16:1010-1016.

56. Trumble TE, Culp RW, Hanel DP, Geissler WB, Berger RA: Intra-articular fractures of the distal aspect of the radius. *Instr Course Lect* 1999;48:465-480.

57. Agee JM: External fixation: Technical advances based upon multiplanar ligamentotaxis. *Orthop Clin North Am* 1993;24:265-274.

58. Markiewitz AD, Gellman H: Five-pin external fixation and early range of motion for distal radius fractures. *Orthop Clin North Am* 2001;32:329-335.

59. Wolfe SW, Swigart CR, Grauer J, Slade JF III, Panjabi MM: Augmented external fixation of distal radius fractures: A biomechanical analysis. *J Hand Surg [Am]* 1998; 23:127-134.

60. Wolfe SW, Austin G, Lorence M, Swigart CR, Panjabi MM: A biomechanical comparison of different wrist external fixators with and without K-wire augmentation. *J Hand Surg [Am]* 1999:24: 516-524.

61. Braun RM, Gellman H: Dorsal pin placement and external fixation for correction of dorsal tilt in fractures of the distal radius. *J Hand Surg [Am]*1994;19:653-655.

62. Wolfe SW, Pike L, Slade JF III, Katz LD: Augmentation of distal radius fracture fixation with coralline hydroxyapatite bone graft substitute. *J Hand Surg [Am]* 1999;24:816-827.

63. Sakano H, Koshino T, Takeuchi R, Sakai N, Saito T: Treatment of the unstable distal radius fracture with external fixation and a hydroxyapatite spacer. *J Hand Surg [Am]* 2001;26:923-930.

64. Cassidy C, Jupiter JB, Cohen M, et al: Norian SRS cement compared with conventional fixation in distal radial fractures: A randomized study. *J Bone Joint Surg Am* 2003;85:2127-2137.

65. Axelrod T, Paley D, Green J, McMurtry RY: Limited open reduction of the lunate facet in comminuted intra-articular fractures of the distal radius. *J Hand Surg [Am]* 1988;13:372-377.

66. Fernandez DL, Geissler WB: Treatment of displaced articular fractures of the radius. *J Hand Surg [Am]* 1991;16:375-384.

67. Melone CP Jr: Articular fractures of the distal radius. *Orthop Clin North Am* 1984;15:217-236.

68. McQueen MM, Caspers J: Colles' fracture: Does the anatomical result affect the final function? *J Bone Joint Surg Br* 1988;70:649-651.

69. Boyd LG, Home JG: The outcome of fractures of the distal radius in young adults. *Injury* 1988;19:97-100.

70. Knirk JL, Jupiter JB: Intra-articular fractures of the distal end of the radius in young adults. *J Bone Joint Surg Am* 1986;68:647-659.

71. Missakian ML, Cooney WP, Amadio PC, Glidwell PA: Open reduction and internal fixation for distal radius fractures. *J Hand Surg [Am]* 1992;17:745-755.

72. Axelrod TS, McMurtry RY: Open reduction and internal fixation of comminuted, intraarticular fractures of the distal radius. *J Hand Surg [Am]* 1990;15:1-11.

73. Hove LM, Nilsen PT, Fumes D, et al: Open reduction and internal fixation of displaced intraarticular fractures of the distal radius: 31 patients followed for 3-7 years. *Acta Orthop Scand* 1997; 68:59-63.

74. Ring D: Intra-articular fractures of the distal radius. *J Am Soc Surg Hand* 2002;2:60-77.

75. Jupiter JB, Fernandez DL, Toh CL, Fellman T, Ring D: Operative

treatment of volar intra-articular fractures of the distal end of the radius. *J Bone Joint Surg Am* 1996;78:1817-1828.

76. Hastings H II, Leibovic SJ: Indications and techniques of open reduction: Internal fixation of distal radius fractures. *Orthop Clin North Am* 1993;24:309-326.

77. Jupiter JB, Ring D, Weitzel PP: Surgical treatment of redisplaced fractures of the distal radius in patients older than 60 years. *J Hand Surg [Am]* 2002;27:714-723.

78. Orbay JL: The treatment of unstable distal radius fractures with volar fixation. *Hand Surg* 2000;5:103-112.

79. Salter RB, Simmonds DF, Malcolm BW, et al: The biological effect of continuous passive motion on the healing of full-thickness defects in articular cartilage: An experimental investigation in the rabibt. *J Bone Joint Surg Am* 1980;62:1232-1351.

80. Osada D, Viegas SF, Shah MA, Morris RF, Patterson RM: Comparison of different distal radius dorsal and volar fracture fixation plates: A biomechanical study. *J Hand Surg [Am]* 2003;28:94-104.

81. Ring D, Jupiter JB, Grennwald J, Buchler U, Hastings H III: Prospective multicenter trial of a plate for dorsal fixation of distal radius fractures. *J Hand Surg [Am]* 1997;22:777-784.

82. Ring D, Jupiter JB: Dorsal fixation of the distal radius using the pi plate. *Atlas Hand Clin* 1997;2: 25-44.

83. Hove LM: Delayed rupture of the thumb extensor tendon: A 5-year study of 18 consecutive cases. *Acta Orthop Scand* 1994;65:199-203.

84. Campbell DA: Open reduction and internal fixation of intra articular and unstable fractures of the distal radius using the AO distal radius plate. *J Hand Surg [Br]* 2000;25:528-534.

85. Kambouroglou GK, Axelrod TS:

Complications of the AO/ASIF titanium distal radius plate system (pi plate) in internal fixation of the distal radius: A brief report. *J Hand Surg [Am]* 1998;23:737-741.

86. Rozental TD, Beredjiklian PK, Bozentka DJ: Functional outcome and complications following two types of dorsal plating for unstable fractures of the distal part of the radius. *J Bone Joint Surg Am* 2003;85:1956-1960.

87. Lowry KJ, Gainor BJ, Hoskins JS: Extensor tendon rupture secondary to the AO/ASIF titanium distal radius plate without associated plate failure: A case report. *Am J Orthop* 2000;29:789-791.

88. Chiang PP, Roach S, Baratz ME: Failure of a retinacular flap to prevent dorsal wrist pain after titanium pi plate fixation of distal radius fractures. *J Hand Surg [Am]* 2002;27:724-728.

89. Lucas GL, Fejfar ST: Complications in internal fixation of the distal radius. *J Hand Surg [Am]* 1998;23:1117.

90. Nunley JA, Rowan PR: Delayed rupture of the flexor pollicis longus tendon after inappropriate placement of the pi plate on the volar surface of the distal radius. *J Hand Surg [Am]*1999;24:1279-1280.

91. Schnur DP, Chang B: Extensor tendon rupture after internal fixation of a distal radius fracture using a dorsally placed AO/ASIF titanium pi plate. *Ann Plast Surg* 2000;44:564-566.

92. Kamano M, Honda Y, Kazuki K, Yasuda M: Palmar plating for dorsally displaced fractures of the distal radius. *Clin Orthop* 2002; 397:403-408.

93. Orbay JL, Fernandez DL: Volar fixation for dorsally displaced fractures of the distal radius: A preliminary report. *J Hand Surg [Am]* 2002;27:205-215.

94. Keating JF, Court-Brown CM, McQueen MM: Internal fixation

of volar-displaced distal radial fractures. *J Bone Joint Surg Br* 1994;76:401-405.

95. Orbay JL, Fernandez DL: Volar fixed-angle plate fixation for unstable distal radius fractures in the elderly patient. *J Hand Surg [Am]* 2004;29:96-102.

96. Boyer MI, Korcek KJ, Gelberman RH, Gilula LA, Ditsios K, Evanoff BA: Anatomic tilt x-rays of the distal radius: An ex vivo analysis of surgical fixation. *J Hand Surg [Am]* 2004;29:116-122.

97. Wolfe SW, Easterling KJ, Yoo HH: Arthroscopic-assisted reduction of distal radius fractures. *Arthroscopy* 1995;11:706-714.

98. Geissler WB, Freeland AE, Savoie FH, McIntyre LW, Whipple TL: Intracarpal soft-tissue lesions associated with an intra-articular fracture of the distal end of the radius. *J Bone Joint Surg Am* 1996;78:357-365.

99. Arrington ED, Smith WJ, Chambers HG, Bucknall AL, Davino NA: Complications of iliac crest bone graft harvesting. *Clin Orthop* 1996;329:300-309.

100. Schmalholz A: Bone cement for redislocated Colles' fracture: A prospective comparison with closed treatment. *Acta Orthop Scand* 1989;60:212-217.

101. Sanchez-Sotelo J, Munuera L, Madero R: Treatment of fractures of the distal radius with a remodellable bone cement: A prospective, randomised study using Norian SRS. *J Bone Joint Surg Br* 2000;82:856-863.

102. Kopylov P, Runnqvist K, Jonsson K, Aspenberg P: Norian SRS versus external fixation in redisplaced distal radial fractures: A randomized study in 40 patients. *Acta Orthop Scand* 1999;70:1-5.

103. Ladd AL, Pliam NB: Use of bone-graft substitutes in distal radius fractures. *J Am Acad Orthop Surg* 1999;7:279-290.

Chapter 7

ASSOCIATED INJURIES

Peter J. Ronchetti, MD

CASE PRESENTATION

A 67-year-old right-handed woman with a history of diabetes mellitus fell on the ice, injuring her right wrist. Examination in the emergency department revealed an open wound on the volar ulnar aspect of the wrist and paresthesias in the median nerve distribution, but her ulnar sensation and vascular status were normal. Radiographs showed a comminuted intra-articular distal radius fracture with both dorsal and volar comminution and a scaphoid fracture (**Figure 1**). Initial treatment consisted of irrigation and débridement in the operating room followed by application of a splint. She was then referred for definitive fracture fixation.

Physical examination at referral evaluation revealed gross swelling at the wrist with altered static two-point discrimination in the distribution of the median nerve. She had poor range of motion (ROM) in her fingers and signs of acute carpal tunnel syndrome but no signs of infection.

DISCUSSION
Compartment Syndrome and Median Nerve Dysfunction

Nerve injuries commonly occur with distal radius fractures. The injury itself may produce an acute compression of the median, ulnar, and/or radial sensory nerves. The median nerve is most commonly affected in acute compression after distal radius fractures and is the most serious sequela.[1-4] Carpal tunnel release can be performed urgently or at the time of surgical fixation, depending on the severity of the patient's symptoms. Initial treatment may lead to an acute compression of the nerve, or posttreatment swelling may be a cause of neurologic dysfunction. Therefore, careful neurologic examination is mandatory in these patients.

Natural History

The first step in treatment of a patient with documented neurologic dysfunction is fracture reduction and splinting or casting. Symptoms generally improve within 24 to 48 hours, but if they do not or if they become worse, then loosening of the cast or splint may relieve the symptoms. If symptoms persist despite

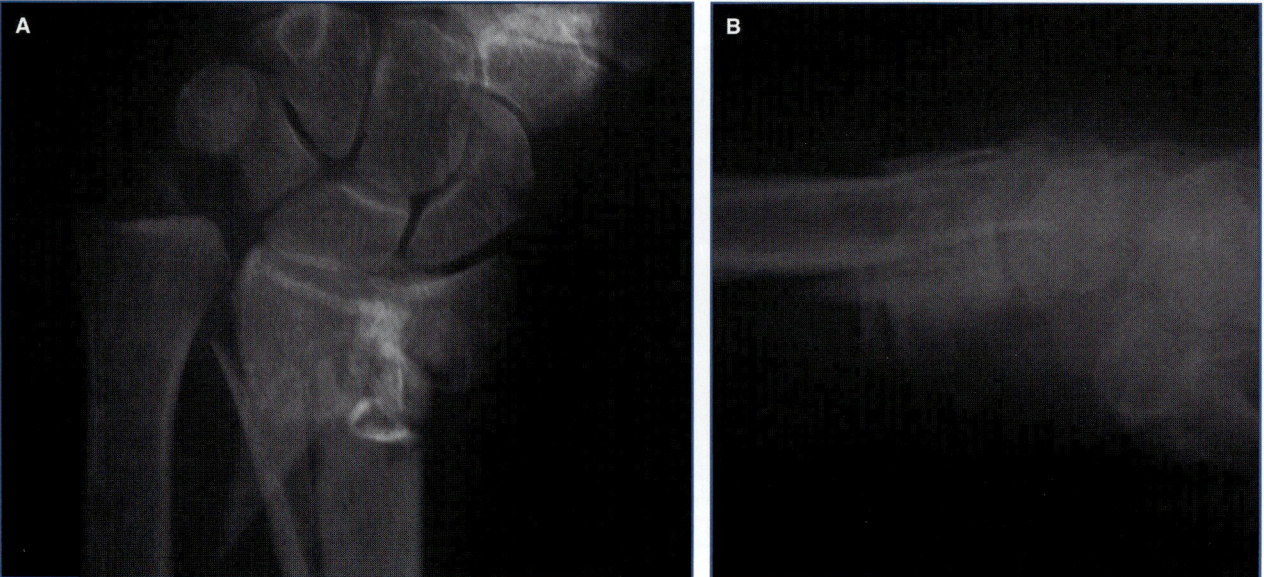

Figure 1 PA **(A)** and lateral **(B)** preoperative radiographs.

loosening or if the patient is unresponsive, then measurement of compartment pressure or surgical decompression may be indicated. I prefer the latter. Surgical decompression of the involved nerve usually is appropriate in these situations; there is very little surgical risk with decompression, but if increased nerve pressure is not treated, the result can be devastating. Mini-open techniques should be avoided in this situation; complete decompression of the involved nerve is required.[1]

Splinting and casting always should be done in a position that prevents compression. Therefore, extremes of flexion and extension must be avoided. Placing the wrist in neutral causes the least pressure in the carpal canal.[5] If fracture reduction can be maintained only in an extreme of either flexion or extension, the fracture is probably best treated surgically.

Compartment syndrome following distal radius fractures occurs most commonly in the volar compartment of the forearm with extension into the carpal tunnel.[6] Predisposing factors are high-energy fractures with significant displacement and soft-tissue injury. Release of both the volar forearm compartment and the carpal tunnel is indicated in these situations. Release of the dorsal forearm compartment is indicated if it remains tense after release of the volar compartment. In a crushing injury, a compartment

syndrome can also develop in the hand. Release of the hand compartments is indicated in these situations. Ten hand compartments may require release: four dorsal interosseous (IO), three volar IO, adductor pollicis, thenar, and hypothenar compartments.

Technique

A two- or three-incision technique can be used to release the IO compartments. I prefer the former. Two dorsal longitudinal incisions are made along the line of the index and ring finger metacarpals (**Figure 2, A**). The first and second dorsal IO compartments can be opened through the incision centered over the index metacarpal. By proceeding deep to the first dorsal IO compartment, the adductor pollicis compartment will be released, and the first palmar IO compartment can be released deep to the second dorsal IO compartment. Through the ring finger metacarpal incision, the third and fourth dorsal IO muscles can be released. Proceeding deep to each of these muscles allows release of the second and third palmar IO compartments. Additional incisions are required to release the thenar and hypothenar compartments (**Figure 2, B**). An additional incision longitudinally radial to the thumb metacarpal allows release of the thenar compartment, and a fourth incision ulnar to the small finger metacar-

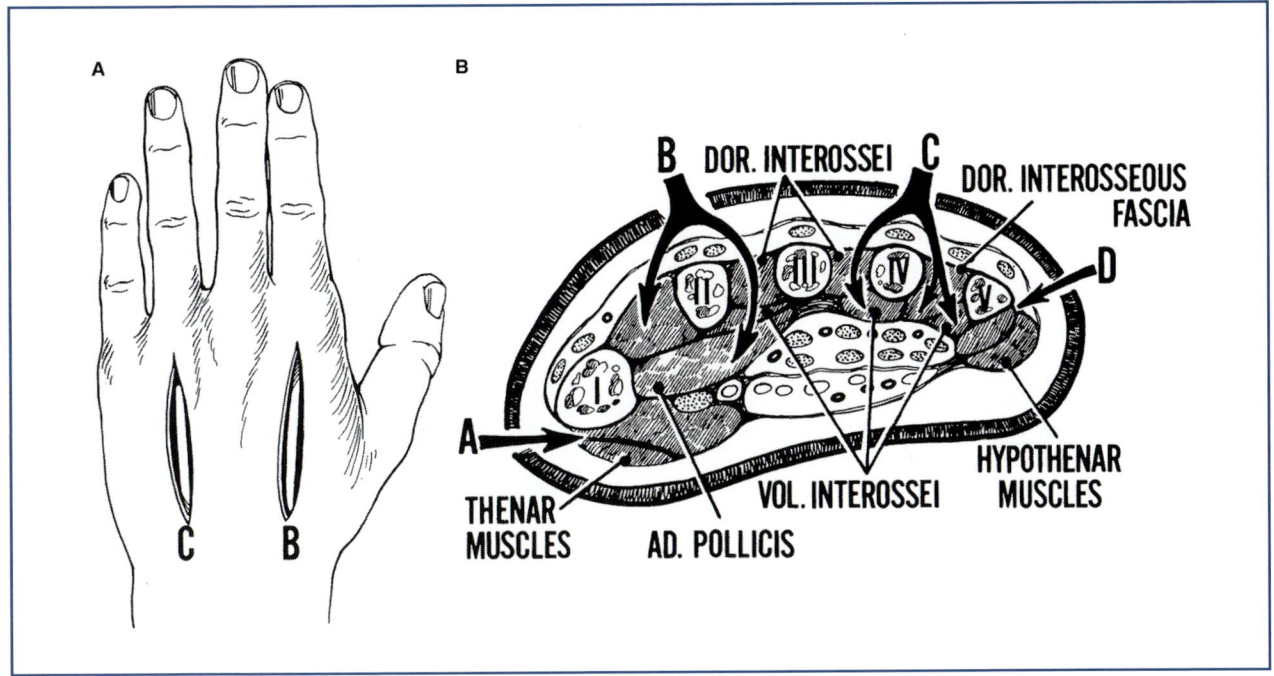

Figure 2 A, Dorsal incisions for hand compartment releases. **B,** Direction of axial plane dissection to release dorsal and volar interosseous compartments (B, C), thenar compartment (A), and hypothenar compartment (D). (Reproduced with permission from Rowland SA: Fasciotomy: The treatment of compartment syndrome, in Green DP, Hotchkiss RN, Pederson WC (eds): *Green's Operative Hand Surgery*, ed 4. Philadelphia, PA, Churchill Livingstone, 1999, pp 689-710.)

pal allows release of the hypothenar compartment. These incisions can be used to release all 10 hand compartments. These wounds usually are left open initially until the acute compression has resolved, then they are skin grafted or closed secondarily.[6]

Release of the volar forearm compartment and carpal tunnel can be done through one large incision that begins at the carpal tunnel and curves ulnar to radial at the level of the middle third of the forearm. The incision curves radially to the proximal third of the forearm, then it curves back ulnarly to end ulnar to the biceps tendon and proximal to the elbow flexion crease. The interval between the flexor digitorum superficialis and the flexor digitorum profundus must be decompressed because this is the site of median nerve compression. Proximally, the median nerve must be released between the two heads of the pronator teres, the superficialis arch, and the lacertus fibrosis. The wounds are left open for later coverage with a skin graft or direct closure if swelling has subsided.[6]

This extensile approach to the forearm also allows visualization of the radial and ulnar arteries if a vascular injury is suspected. If an arterial injury is found, primary repair or reversed vein grafting can be performed. Loupe magnification or a microscope typically is needed to perform these anastomoses.

Anticipation is the key to identifying these injuries. Surgical decompression adds little time to surgical treatment of the high-energy distal radius injury.

Digital Stiffness

If digital stiffness develops in the weeks to months after fracture healing, patients commonly are referred to a hand specialist. To prevent stiffness from developing, a number of steps must be taken during treatment. First, the distal palmar crease must be visible when either a cast or splint is applied to allow unrestricted digital flexion at the metacarpophalangeal (MCP) joints. Second, finger exercises are required five times a day to maintain mobility in the MCP and proximal and distal interphalangeal (IP) joints. These exercises also help with swelling and greatly improve the patient's function. A patient who is noncompliant or cannot perform the exercises because of associated injuries requires supervised hand therapy.

Patients must be advised that the exercises will not prevent fracture healing. Even if the wrist does not function well, if the fingers are free and mobile the patient will be able to perform most activities. These exercises can start immediately because all patients are instructed on them in the recovery room. Both composite exercises (ie, making a fist) and joint isolation exercises for the MCP and proximal and distal IP joints are taught. These exercises are especially critical in elderly patients who may have preexisting osteoarthritis that can make normal function in the fingers difficult to achieve.

An especially difficult problem is severe stiffness in the patient who is placed in an external fixator. This stiffness often is related to overdistraction of the carpus. Therefore, the radiographs of these patients must be examined closely following fixator placement to ensure that the carpus is not distracted from the distal radius. Remember that fracture reduction is a combination of gentle distraction and volar translation of the carpus with respect to the distal radius. Patients can be sent to supervised hand therapy in the first postoperative days to ensure that they are doing the exercises properly.

Other Fractures

The most common fracture associated with injury to the distal radius is the ulnar styloid fracture. Although most ulnar styloid fractures can be treated nonsurgically, careful assessment of the radiographs will identify those that require surgical fixation. Using the AO classification for distal ulna fractures, which divides them into six types, helps identify those that need to be treated surgically.[7] The ulnar styloid is involved in the first three types. Both type 1 (triangular fibrocartilage complex [TFCC] avulsion) and 2B (basistyloid fractures) require surgical fixation; small distal fractures of the styloid (type 2A) do not.

A surgical approach between the flexor carpi ulnaris and extensor carpi ulnaris, with care to protect the dorsal sensory branch of the ulnar nerve, can be used to expose the fracture.[8] The fracture is usually

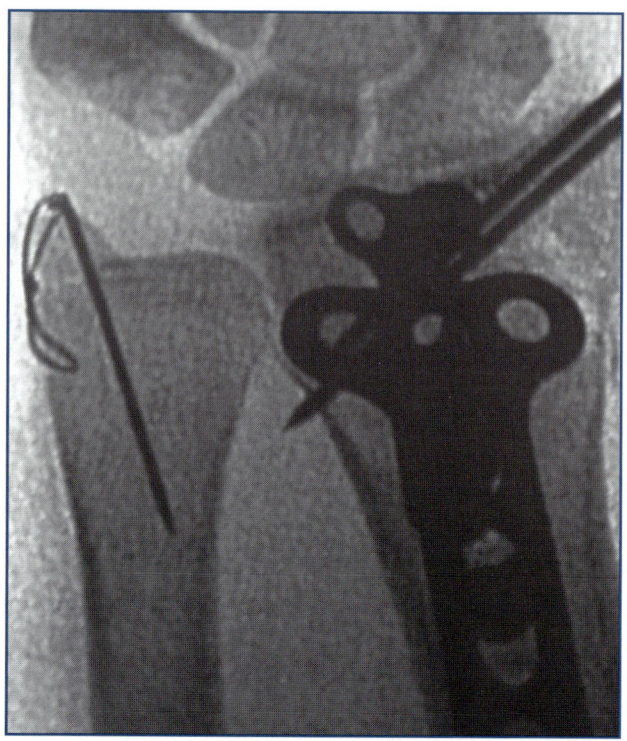

Figure 3 Example of ulnar styloid fixation. A 0.045-in K-wire is placed obliquely through the distal fragment and into the ulna. Then a 26-gauge wire is used in a tension band fashion to provide secure anatomic fixation.

readily visualized; however, the ulnar styloid often is smaller than it appears on radiographs. I prefer provisional fixation using a 0.035-in Kirschner wire (K-wire) as a joystick to reduce the fracture under fluoroscopic guidance. The K-wire must be driven almost vertically to ensure that it catches both the styloid fragment and the ulna. A hole is then drilled transversely proximal to the fracture site with a 0.045-in K-wire. The 26-gauge wire is placed around the vertical K-wire and then it is crossed and placed through the hole in the ulna. It is then tensioned using a heavy needle driver. The wire breaks easily if it is overtightened (**Figure 3**).

Examining the patient under anesthesia also will help in decision making. Patients should be evaluated for distal radioulnar joint instability, which should be compared with the opposite normal side. A large TFCC avulsion can create instability that is best treated with open repair (type 1).[8,9]

High-energy fractures can cause other bony lesions in the carpus. Careful scrutiny of the radiographs will reveal fractures, and these fractures also should be treated surgically using the fixation of the surgeon's choice. It is best to perform the distal radius fixation first and then proceed to the carpal injuries.

Scaphoid fractures are often present in high-energy distal radius fractures. Stable fixation can be achieved with percutaneous pins or screw fixation. The pins can be placed either dorsally or volarly but should exit volarly when appropriate reduction has been obtained. Screw fixation also can be obtained with either a dorsal or volar approach. Paramount to screw fixation of the scaphoid is ensuring accurate central screw placement, which provides the greatest strength. Variable pitch screws also have been shown to be superior in strength.[10]

Arthroscopy and Ligament Injuries

Arthroscopy has a therapeutic role in the treatment of intra-articular distal radius fractures.[11] Arthroscopy provides a means to evaluate articular reconstruction following fracture and identify intra-articular soft-tissue injuries. However, certain fractures are not amenable to arthroscopic-assisted treatment, particularly those with significant articular comminution, because fluid extravasation is a problem in these fractures. Fractures with several large articular pieces are ideal because they can be readily visualized with the arthroscope. At least 48 to 72 hours should elapse from the time of the fracture to consider arthroscopic treatment. The appropriate time is 3 to 7 days from the time of injury. Contraindications to arthroscopic treatment include open fractures and fractures associated with a compartment syndrome.[12]

Increased use of arthroscopy for reduction and fixation has revealed a high percentage of patients with soft-tissue derangements following fracture. Geissler and associates[13] reported on a cohort of patients, 68% of whom had an associated intracarpal soft-tissue injury with an intra-articular fracture of the distal radius. Several factors aided in the diagnosis. The lunate facet is almost always involved in the fracture. Most common injuries were TFCC tears, scapholunate (SL) ligament tears, and lunotriquetral (LT) ligament tears. Large TFCC injuries are best treated with direct repair; SL and LT ligament injuries can be treated with open repair and pinning.[13,14]

The axial scaphoid shift sign is a helpful radiographic parameter.[15] With traction placed on the wrist through finger traps, the relationship between the scaphoid and the lunate should be carefully assessed. In acute SL disruptions, there will be asymmetry between the scaphoid and the lunate so that the proximal pole of the scaphoid appears more distal than normal. This shift breaks Gilula's arc and is a sign of SL disruption.

Radial styloid fractures also should be carefully evaluated for a possible associated SL ligament injury. A transradial perilunate dislocation can be present and may be overlooked.

Arthroscopy is performed in the standard fashion with the patient's hand placed in the traction device. A 3-4 portal is established followed by a 6U outflow portal (**Figure 4**). Either the 3-4 or 1-2 portals (or both) can be used. The clot must be irrigated from the fracture site and closed reduction performed. Joysticks often are helpful to manipulate the fracture fragments into an anatomic position. Visualization of the fracture fragments will aid in the accuracy of reduction. The wrist also can be examined for any ligament injuries.

Open repair of SL or LT ligament injuries is challenging. I prefer a dorsal longitudinal approach with an anatomic capsular incision.[16] The capsular incision is a triangularly shaped, radially based flap along the line of the dorsoradiocarpal and dorsal intercarpal ligaments. Once this flap of capsule is raised, the SL and LT ligament injuries can be well visualized. The type of repair depends on the type of tear. The most important part of the SL ligament is its dorsal portion; therefore, this is the critical area in which to obtain a strong repair. Midsubstance tears can be directly repaired with a No. 3-0 nonabsorbable suture. Most tears occur off of the scaphoid, and several approaches can be used. Suture anchors placed in the scaphoid or lunate can be used to reattach the ligament. Typically, the scaphoid is reduced and pinned to the capitate with a 0.045-in K-wire. Next, the lunate is reduced, and two divergent SL pins are placed. Following this step, the anchors, preferably two, can be placed and the sutures looped in a mattress form through the ligament stump and tied down. Alternatively, bone tunnels can be placed from the ligament insertion through the scaphoid to its waist. Nonabsorbable suture can then be placed through the liga-

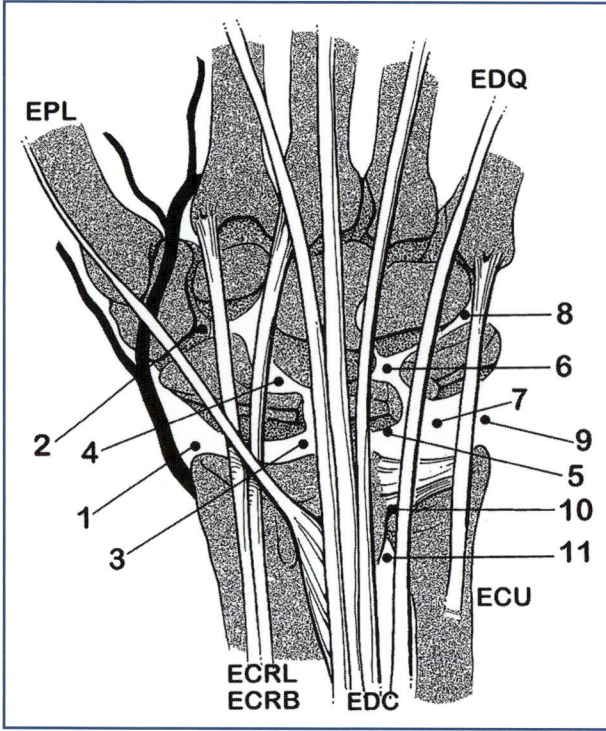

Figure 4 Portals used for wrist arthroscopy. The 3-4 portal (3), the 4-5 portal (5), the 1-2 portal (1), and the 6 U portal (9), which is named 6 U because it is ulnar to the extensor carpi ulnaris tendon. (Reproduced with permission from Poehling GG, Ruch DS: Wrist arthroscopy: Anatomy and diagnosis, in Green DP, Hotchkiss RN, Pederson WC (eds): *Green's Operative Hand Surgery*, ed 4. Philadelphia, PA, Churchill Livingstone, 1999, pp 192-199.)

ment stump and, with the aid of straight needles, these sutures can be passed through the holes and tied.[17]

The anatomic capsular incision is then closed, and the pins are either cut beneath the skin or left out. Pins typically are left in place for 8 weeks provided no pin tract infections occur. Total time of immobilization varies, but usually it is close to 3 months.

Tendon Problems

Tendon problems that can occur in association with a distal radius fracture include tendon adhesions, entrapment within the fracture site, tenosynovitis, laceration, and rupture.[1,3,4]

Early ROM exercises can prevent or decrease the

severity of tendon adhesions. Virtually all patients with a distal radius fracture require supervised hand therapy to ensure that they understand both the importance of the exercises and how to perform them. Patients must also understand that elevation of the affected extremity is critical in the first week following injury. Elevation decreases swelling and eases the discomfort of ROM exercises. All of my patients are sent home with an arm elevation pillow, regardless of treatment (ie, cast or surgery).

Tendon entrapment within the fracture site is a rare occurrence. When a fracture cannot be reduced and digital ROM is poor, or there is loss of the normal tenodesis effect with flexion and extension of the wrist, possible tendon entrapment should be suspected. An inadequate reduction should not be confused with a persistent irreducible fracture. If the patient is under adequate anesthesia, all fractures can be reduced to some degree. Fractures that show persistent significant displacement require open reduction and removal of the incarcerated tendon from the fracture site. Any of the digital flexor tendons can be involved; however, the extensor carpi ulnaris and the extensor digiti quinti proprius are most commonly involved on the extensor surface.

Late tendon attrition is not uncommon: it occurs in patients whose fractures are not severely displaced, up to weeks or years after the initial injury. The extensor pollicis longus (EPL) is usually involved.[1,3,4] The pathologic site is at Lister's tubercle where a mini compartment syndrome occurs, resulting in loss of normal tendon blood flow and ultimately attritional rupture. Displaced fracture fragments also can fray the tendon to the point at which it ruptures. Direct repair is not advised. These problems are best handled by a tendon transfer, the most popular of which is an extensor indicis proprius (EIP) to EPL transfer. Other donors include the palmaris longus, the extensor digiti quinti proprius, and the flexor digitorum superficialis from the ring finger.

The EIP to EPL transfer is very straightforward (**Figure 5**). Three incisions are necessary. A transverse incision just proximal to the MCP joint extension crease of the index finger is made to expose the EIP tendon. The EIP tendon is always ulnar to the extensor digitorum communis tendon to the index finger. The EIP is transected just proximal to the MCP joint. Next, a longitudinal incision is made between the third and fourth extensor compartments at the distal

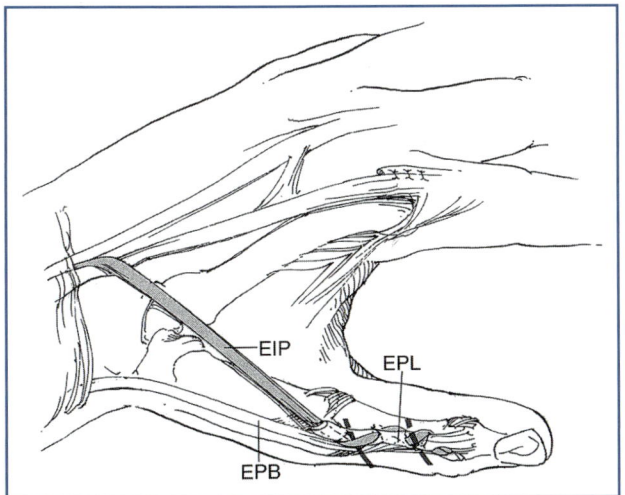

Figure 5 EIP to EPL tendon transfer. The EIP is harvested over the index finger and rerouted from the fourth extensor compartment to the remaining EPL tendon. It is then weaved through the EPL tendon and sutured using nonabsorbable sutures. (Reproduced with permission from Perlic DC: Extensor radius proprius transfer for EPL rupture, in Blair WF (ed): *Techniques in Hand Surgery.* Baltimore, MD, Williams & Wilkins, 1996, pp 649-653.)

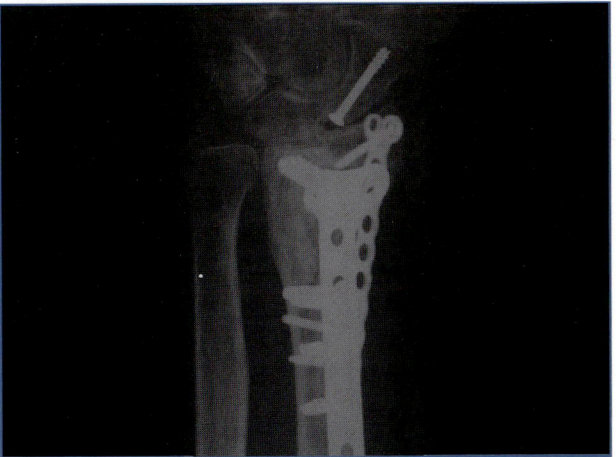

Figure 6 PA postoperative radiograph.

retinaculum of the EIP. The distal edge of the EPL can be retrieved through this incision and the EIP located. The attritional area of the tendon should be excised. Traction is placed on the EIP tendon, and it is delivered into the proximal wound. A third incision (I prefer a chevron type) is made over the thumb metacarpal. A subcutaneous tunnel is then made using a small curved hemostat, and the EIP is routed from the distal retinaculum to the dorsum of the thumb metacarpal. The EIP is then weaved into the EPL with a tendon weaver. With the wrist in 30° of extension and the thumb in full extension, the transfer is sutured in place with a No. 3-0 nonabsorbable suture. In a test of the transfer, wrist flexion should result in thumb extension dorsal to the plane of the palm, and wrist extension should allow passive abduction and opposition of the thumb. This transfer should be made a little tight because it will tend to stretch with time and hand therapy. The thumb typically is held in a thumb spica splint or cast for 4 weeks, with the thumb held in opposition, and then active and passive motion of the thumb is begun. Patients do very well after this transfer.[18]

Miscellaneous Injuries
Dupuytren's Contracture

Any injury to the wrist or hand can cause a Dupuytren's flare in a patient predisposed to Dupuytren's disease. Aggressive hand therapy and extension splinting may be necessary. Surgical treatment of the Dupuytren's contracture should not be considered until the fracture has healed, and all wounds have become quiescent.[1,3]

Vascular Injury

Vascular injury is uncommon but can occur from fracture fragments or a penetrating injury. Careful preoperative vascular examination and repair of the injured vessels is mandatory. If a vascular injury is suspected, a hand surgeon should assist in the vascular repair.

MANAGEMENT AND OUTCOME SUMMARY

The patient was taken to the operating room for open reduction and internal fixation of the radius using two plates, open reduction and internal fixation of the scaphoid, and open carpal tunnel release. The postoperative image is shown in **Figure 6**. Postoperatively, the patient's fractures healed, and she was extremely pleased with her ROM. She had a residual deficit in the sensation of the median nerve, but her motor function was excellent. Overall she had a very good result from a highly comminuted injury.

Several points can be learned from this case. Even if definitive fixation is not planned at the time of initial irrigation and débridement, preliminary reduction should be performed. If this reduction fails to reasonably align the fracture fragments, then application of a bridging external fixator is appropriate. Clearly the patient had signs and symptoms of carpal tunnel syndrome at initial presentation; yet, despite a trip to the operating room, no carpal tunnel release was performed.

Definitive fracture fixation does not have to occur at initial presentation. External fixation with appropriate nerve decompression allows swelling to subside and provides the treating surgeon a chance to best plan surgical treatment.

The key to prevention of any impending complication is anticipation. Most complications can be prevented if time is taken to evaluate each injury individually. All distal radius fractures have individual characteristics. Each fracture should be addressed systematically so that the most appropriate treatment can be rendered. A detailed patient history, including identifying the dominant hand, a careful neurologic examination, and critical review of the radiographs, is very important. Problems most often arise when the surgeon fails to do the latter two.

REFERENCES

1. Fernandez D, Jupiter J: Early complications, in Fernandez D, Jupiter J (eds): *Fractures of the Distal Radius*. New York, NY, Springer-Verlag, 1996, pp 317-337.

2. Jupiter J: Fractures of the distal end of the radius. *J Bone Joint Surg Am* 1991;73:461-469.

3. Kozin S, Wood M: Early soft-tissue complications after fractures of the distal part of the radius. *J Bone Joint Surg Am* 1993;75:144-153.

4. Cooney W, Dobyns J, Linscheid R: Complications of Colles' fractures. *J Bone Joint Surg Am* 1980;62:613-619.

5. Gelberman R, Szabo R, Mortensen W: Carpal tunnel pressures and wrist position in patients with Colles' fractures. *J Trauma* 1984;24:747-749.

6. Rowland S: Fasciotomy: The treatment of compartment syndrome, in Green DP, Hotchkiss RN, Pederson WP (eds): *Green's Operative Hand Surgery*, ed 4. Philadelphia, PA, Churchill Livingstone, 1999, pp 689-710.

7. McCallister W, Trumble T: Introduction to section II: Distal radius fractures and overview and algorithms for treatment, in Trumble TE (ed): *Hand Surgery Update 3*. Rosemont, IL, American Society for Surgery of the Hand, 2003, pp 67-82.

8. Cooney W: Tears of the triangular fibrocartilage of the wrist, in Cooney W, Linscheid R, Dobyns J (eds): *The Wrist: Diagnosis and Operative Treatment*. St. Louis, MO, Mosby, 1998, pp 710-742.

9. Cooney W: Fractures of the distal radius, in Cooney W, Linscheid R, Dobyns J (eds): *The Wrist: Diagnosis and Operative Treatment*. St. Louis, MO, Mosby, 1998, pp 310-355.

10. Knoll V, Trumble T: Scaphoid fractures and nonunion, in Trumble TE (ed): *Hand Surgery Update 3*. Rosemont, IL, American Society for Surgery of the Hand, 2003, pp 161-173.

11. Hanel D: Treatment of intra-articular fractures, in Trumble TE (ed): *Hand Surgery Update 3*. Rosemont, IL, American Society for Surgery of the Hand, 2003, pp 105-121.

12. Fernandez D, Palmer A: Fractures of the distal radius, in Green D (ed): *Green's Operative Hand Surgery*, ed 4. Philadelphia, PA, Churchill Livingstone, 1999, pp 929-985.

13. Geissler W, Freeland A, Savoie FH, McIntyre LW, Whipple TL: Intracarpal soft-tissue lesions associated with an intra-articular fracture of the distal end of the radius. *J Bone Joint Surg Am* 1996;78:357-365.

14. Smith D, Henry M: Comprehensive management of soft-tissue injuries associated with distal radius fractures. *J Am Soc Surg Hand* 2002;2:153-164.

15. Fernandez D, Jupiter J: Combined fractures of the distal radius: Type V, in Fernandez D, Jupiter J (eds): *Fractures of the Distal Radius*. New York, NY, Springer-Verlag, 1996, pp 235-261.

16. Ruby L: Arthrotomy, in Cooney W, Linscheid R, Dobyns J (eds): *The Wrist: Diagnosis and Operative Treatment*. St. Louis, MO, Mosby, 1998, pp 126-168.

17. Wolfe S: Scapholunate instability. *J Am Soc Surg Hand* 2001;1:45-60.

18. Smith R: Tendon transfers following trauma or ischemic necrosis, in Smith RJ (ed): *Tendon Transfers of the Hand and Forearm*. Boston, MA, Little, Brown, 1987, pp 263-285.

INDEX